Get Throug~~h Radiology~~ for the MRCS and the FRCS

An essential handbook that covers the radiological findings of all the common surgical conditions. Candidates preparing for the MRCS or FRCS (in General Surgery) exams will find this indispensable guide will prepare them for a wide range of questions, including rare and obscure examples that are not found elsewhere.

Radiological findings are presented according to systems such as colorectal, upper GI and HPB, urology, emergency surgery and others. Each chapter describes the use of radiological modalities in different clinical scenarios and includes figures illustrating the defining characteristics of common clinical scenarios.

The clear and illustrated content provides the knowledge required to answer what would otherwise be some of the most difficult questions in postgraduate surgical examinations. It is also a practical reference book that can be kept at hand to inform ward rounds and multidisciplinary team meetings. MRCS and FRCS exam candidates are expected to have a knowledge of radiological findings for all surgical conditions, and this concise guide will ensure that candidates are well prepared to answer questions accurately and with confidence.

Miss. Zaynab Jawad is a Consultant General Surgeon based at Ealing Hospital, London North West University Healthcare Trust. She has an interest in laparoscopic and benign upper gastrointestinal and hepatobiliary surgery. She studied medicine at Corpus Christi College, Cambridge and Imperial College London, graduating with distinction. She completed her surgical training in North West London, during which time she completed a PhD in nanotechnology from the Department of Engineering at Imperial College London. She has authored multiple peer-reviewed papers, including those in high-impact journals.

Dr Susan Jawad is a Consultant Radiologist based at University College London Hospitals (UCLH), where she sub-specialises in head and neck radiology and is the Trust Lead for MRI. She graduated in medicine with distinction from Imperial College London and trained in radiology in South West and North Central London. She has lectured nationally and internationally and has authored book chapters as well as several peer-reviewed publications. She is an experienced trainer and supervisor of radiology trainees and also teaches ENT trainees.

GET THROUGH

About the Series

Our bestselling *Get Through* series guides medical postgraduates through the many exams they will need to pass throughout their career, whatever their specialty. Each title is written by authors with recent first-hand experience of the exam, overseen and edited by experts in the field to ensure each question or scenario closely matches the latest examining board guidelines. Detailed explanations and background knowledge provide all you need to know to get through your postgraduate medical examination.

For more information about this series please visit: *https://www.routledge.com/Get-Through/book-series/crcgetthroug*

Get Through Radiology for the MRCS and the FRCS

Zaynab Jawad
MA (Cantab) MBBS MSc PhD FRCS

Susan Jawad
BSc MBBS FRCR

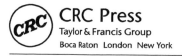

CRC Press
Taylor & Francis Group
Boca Raton London New York

CRC Press is an imprint of the
Taylor & Francis Group, an **informa** business

First edition published 2024
by CRC Press
2385 NW Executive Center Drive, Suite 320, Boca Raton, FL 33431

and by CRC Press
4 Park Square, Milton Park, Abingdon, Oxon, OX14 4RN

CRC Press is an imprint of Taylor & Francis Group, LLC

ISBN: 978-1-032-34903-9 (hbk)
ISBN: 978-1-032-34902-2 (pbk)
ISBN: 978-1-003-32436-2 (ebk)

DOI: 10.1201/9781003324362

Typeset in Sabon
by Apex CoVantage, LLC

With love and affection, we dedicate this book to our parents, who always encouraged us to pay it forward, and to our children, who continue to inspire us.

Contents

Preface

Diagnostic imaging has become a crucial adjunct in the management of patients across the surgical specialties. Due to the massive expansion of imaging across healthcare, the surgeon in training must have a good awareness of the uses of various imaging modalities for surgical conditions and when it is appropriate to request them. There has been a shift in recent years towards much closer multidisciplinary working between surgeons and radiologists, traditionally for oncology cases but more recently also for the management of benign cases, where the imaging is crucial for anatomical delineation, including for potential surgical hazards, which often aid the surgical approach, with undoubted benefits for the patient. Furthermore, the dialogue between the surgeon who has clinical knowledge of the patient and the radiologist who has the expertise to interpret the radiological findings is paramount in deciding the best strategy of care for the patient.

Depending on the clinical setting, radiological reports may not be instantly available; therefore, it may be necessary for the managing surgeon to provisionally scrutinise available imaging themselves, especially in the emergency context.

Get Through Radiology for the MRCS and the FRCS is a concise but comprehensive handbook for surgeons. It is an essential guide that covers the radiological findings of all the common surgical conditions to ensure the candidate has a good idea of the radiological considerations going into the exam and for day-to-day practice. Multiple hints around image interpretation of these conditions are presented. For candidates preparing for the MRCS or FRCS (in General Surgery) exams, this is an indispensable guide that will help in the preparation for those obscure radiology questions that are not covered in any other textbook and that have become a predictable part of the examination, particularly in the written but also in the oral section. It is also a reference book that can be kept at hand to inform ward rounds and multidisciplinary team meetings. In this manner, it will not only be an invaluable resource for medical students and junior surgeons but this text will also have an indispensable use going forward for senior trainees and consultant specialists as a reference guide.

Chapter 1

Radiological Modalities

PLAIN X-RAY FILM AND FLUOROSCOPY

Plain film is still a crucial modality for investigating surgical patients. It can provide a quick radiological assessment of the neck, chest, abdomen and axial and appendicular skeleton. Plain film is mostly utilised in the emergency situation and comes at a relatively low radiological dose, which is an important consideration in younger patients who are more sensitive to the effective dose of radiation.

X-rays are a high-energy, high-frequency form of electromagnetic radiation that are produced by electrons within an X-ray tube. The X-rays pass through the patient and onto a film cassette, which detects the X-rays and produces the image. Dense material, such as bone and metal, absorbs the X-rays and effectively blocks their transmission, thus forming a whiter image as opposed to air and fat, which better transmits the X-rays and form a blacker image. Other forms of soft tissue are depicted in varying tones of grey, depending on their density.

Common surgical conditions still assessed as a first line with plain film are retained foreign bodies, e.g., fishbones in the throat (lateral soft tissue radiograph), trauma (though cases of major trauma are being replaced with CT), suspected perforated viscus (erect chest radiograph and abdominal radiograph) and suspected bowel obstruction.

Fluoroscopy uses X-rays delivered via an image-intensifier system to produce the radiological images, often with the use of barium and or gastrograffin as dense contrast agents to highlight various anatomical lumens and their associated pathologies, for example, fistulas and mural dehiscence.

MAMMOGRAPHY

Mammography utilises dedicated X-ray equipment to image the breast tissue, providing information on the nature of tissues constituting the breast. Typically, two images of each breast are acquired, the craniocaudal (CC) 'top-down' view and the mediolateral oblique (MLO), taken laterally at an

DOI: 10.1201/9781003324362-1

1

angle. Mammography is used in both symptomatic patients who have a lump as well as asymptomatic patients during routine screening. Lesions identified on mammography can be targeted for biopsy using mammography, US or MRI.

ULTRASOUND (US)

US is an incredibly useful modality for assessment of multiple surgical conditions. Unlike CT and plain film, there is no safety concern regarding radiation dose, and compared to MRI, resolution of the anatomical structures and pathological processes can be much better delineated with this modality, especially for musculoskeletal and head and neck conditions. US also has an important use in assessment of the paediatric patient, where plain film and CT may not be considered appropriate as first-line modalities due to the potential harm radiation exposure can cause. Another advantage of US is the ability to perform interventional procedures for diagnosis or treatment under US guidance such as drains, core biopsies and fine needle aspiration (FNA). US is, however, operator dependent; the quality of the imaging produced can differ depending on the experience of the operator; and it is often not available out of hours, in which case an alternative modality will have to be requested, even if US would have ideally been the first line investigation.

Contrast agents can be employed in US, where it is particularly useful for assessment of hepatic and renal lesions and for small and large bowel lesions.

COMPUTED TOMOGRAPHY (CT)

For most surgical conditions, computed tomography (CT) has largely taken over to provide a more accurate and reliable anatomical assessment of the surgical patient.

X-rays are utilised to form a volumetric dataset of images that can be manipulated in the axial, sagittal and coronal as well as oblique planes to scrutinise the volume of the body that has been scanned. Due to its reliance on X-rays, various body tissues, gas and foreign bodies (i.e., metal) have different greyscale appearances that can be quantified with the Hounsfield unit (HU, named after Sir Godfrey Hounsfield, who won the Nobel Prize in Physiology or Medicine for his part in developing CT). HUs are invaluable to establish the nature of the material being examined on a scan: 0 HU is taken as water density, soft tissue measures between 20–80 HUs, bone measures on average between 400–1000 HUs and at the other end of the Hounsfield scale, fat measures between –40 to –100 HUs and air measures around –1000 HUs. Post-processing on a picture archiving and communication system (PACS) can accentuate certain soft tissues by defining the range on HUs that are optimally depicted on the images; these so-called windows can be employed to highlight tissue better, and among others, there are bone, lung, brain and soft tissue windows. In some cases, it is useful to use a certain window to accentuate material in a different part of the body; for example, a lung window can be used in the abdomen to better detect luminal, mural, peritoneal or portal gas.

Iodinated contrast is usually administered prior to the CT at variable intervals depending on the clinical question as different vessels and tissues and their associated pathologies enhance variably at different time intervals since the contrast was administered; therefore, contrast can help identify the nature of the tissue or pathology. Contrast can be water insoluble in the case of barium sulphate or water soluble in the case of gastrograffin. The latter is implemented more in the surgical context due to its absorbability and safety, should there be a confirmed or risk of loss of integrity of the bowel wall. Barium still has an important role in elective fluoroscopic studies, namely barium swallows and meals. Barium enemas are now confined to the radiological archives due to the advent and widespread implementation of colonoscopy and CT colonography (CTC).

As CT uses ionising radiation in the form of X-rays, it may be more suitable to employ other modalities as a first line to minimise the effect of the radiation dose on the patient; for example, a paediatric patient with suspected appendicitis could be examined with US as a first line and CT performed only if there is still diagnostic uncertainty and if the US is inconclusive.

MAGNETIC RESONANCE IMAGING (MRI)

Magnetic resonance imaging (MRI) utilises a strong magnetic field and radiofrequency energy to map the hydrogen (i.e., water and fat) density of different tissues into an image. The appearance of different tissues or materials can be altered if different radiofrequency pulses and gradients are applied to the tissues within the strong magnetic field. These differences result in the generation of different sequences, for example, T1-, T2- and diffusion-weighted imaging (DWI) sequences. Different tissues have different greyscale values in these different sequences, which can help the radiologist identify the nature of a tissue. For example, in the middle ear, fluid in the form of an effusion is as bright as cholesteatoma on a T2 sequence, but cholesteatoma is very bright on DW imaging, much more so than fluid, so using these sequences the radiologist can identify if one or both of these conditions are present. It is the responsibility of the radiologist to decide which sequences are required depending on the clinical question being posed by the surgeon; it is important to do enough sequences to answer the clinical question but to avoid doing superfluous sequences that will inconvenience the patient and reduce the efficiency of the scanner and service. Substances that are attracted by the magnetic field such as gadolinium are known as paramagnetic substances, and these may be given as an intravenous contrast agent to enhance the appearance of certain tissues. MRI has many advantages, such as producing high contrast between tissues, both anatomical and pathological. Another key advantage is that unlike CT, MRI does not use ionising radiation so it is useful in children and pregnant patients in particular. One of the main disadvantages of MRI is that these studies take significantly longer than CT, and the patient needs to remain very still, which is a challenge for some patients, particularly if they are confused. The magnetic field is generated by a permanent magnet surrounding the patient as a bore, which some patients find distressing due to claustrophobia.

POSITRON EMISSION TOMOGRAPHY (PET) SCANNING

During a PET scan, a radioactive material known as a tracer bound to a compound containing glucose (commonly fluorodeoxyglucose, FDG, but other compounds are also used) is injected intravenously. Due to the presence of glucose bound to the radioactive tracer, metabolically active tissues, such as malignancies and inflammatory tissues, readily take up the tracer. The location of the radioactive tracer in the body is detected and a map localising the tracer is produced. Patients will often have a whole-body CT or MRI scan that the radiotracer map can be superimposed on, to better localise the tracer uptake.

RADIONUCLEOTIDE SCANNING

Radiotracers can be administered intravenously or orally to patients. These are in turn taken up by certain tissues more avidly than others, and the anatomical location of these radiotracers are detected by specialist equipment, forming an image. As well as anatomical information, radionucleotide scanning can also be useful to determine how an organ functions, for example, in the case of MAG3 scans, whereby the location as well as the function of the kidneys is determined.

Chapter 2

Emergency Surgery

Imaging plays a crucial role in the management of surgical patients in the emergency setting. Laparotomy was once considered a diagnostic procedure, but this has mostly been replaced by pre-operative computed tomography (CT) scanning to provide diagnostic information prior to going ahead with surgery, both to help in decision making and plan the operative approach. Furthermore, the improvements in resolution and the development and expansion of interventional radiology (IR) have provided less invasive strategies to deal with common presentations such as bleeding and for sepsis control. If it is an option, implementation of IR is usually the preferred approach, particularly in co-morbid patients, as it can reduce morbidity and mortality and thereby improve outcomes in patients who would not otherwise be fit to undergo the knife. The collaboration between surgeon and radiologist is crucial in bringing together the clinical assessment of the patient with the radiological assessment, and it is particularly important in deciding on any clinico-radiological ambiguities.

In this chapter, common surgical emergencies are presented to discuss the preferred imaging modalities and radiological findings in each of the cases.

ACUTE INTESTINAL OBSTRUCTION

Intestinal obstruction accounts for around 10% of acute surgical admissions with more than 70% of cases being due to small bowel obstruction (1). The role of imaging is not only to confirm the presence and location of the obstruction but also assesses the likely cause and, in some cases, imaging can also help detect if there are any associated complications such as bowel ischaemia or perforation. These guide the management of the patient and can also flag up any patients who need urgent surgical intervention. Abdominal X-ray (AXR) is often the first imaging modality used to assess patients presenting with suspected bowel obstruction. These are readily available in emergency departments and are highly useful in detecting the presence of bowel obstruction, with an accuracy of between 50% and 80% (2). With the advent of increased CT scanner capacity, and in some centres where CT

DOI: 10.1201/9781003324362-2

scanners are based in the emergency department, many patients progress immediately to CT, especially in those with a high clinical suspicion and where the anatomical detail will be required for surgical planning (see CT section).

AXR

Abdominal X-rays can provide a lot of information if interpreted adequately. Furthermore, as previously mentioned they are widely available, which is another huge advantage. AXRs can help differentiate large from small bowel obstruction and may detect certain causes such as sigmoid volvulus (see following section). The disadvantages of AXRs are that they cannot detect ischaemic compromise to the small bowel well, and in the context of large bowel obstruction they cannot always detect closed loop obstructions and neither can they differentiate a paralytic ileus or pseudo-obstruction from a mechanical obstruction, which CT is better at differentiating. Absence of dilated large bowel suggests either a mechanical small bowel obstruction or a paralytic ileus (also known as a functional obstruction). It is important to differentiate the two as a paralytic ileus is treated conservatively. This can usually be confirmed on CT abdomen. Similarly, a pseudo-obstruction is seen as dilated large bowel, which may be present to the rectum. Again, this usually needs to be confirmed on CT scan. The presence of air or stool in the rectum goes against bowel obstruction. Erect chest X-ray (CXR) is often requested in conjunction with AXR to exclude a pneumoperitoneum, which may occur if a bowel obstruction is complicated by a perforation.

On abdominal X-ray, small bowel obstruction is characterised by dilated small bowel loops (quantified by a diameter of greater than 3 cm) and paucity of gas within normal sized colonic loops (Figure 2.1).

Large bowel obstruction is seen as dilated large bowel loops (greater than 6 cm) with or without small bowel dilatation (Figure 2.2). Small bowel dilatation may be seen in the presence of an incompetent ileocaecal valve.

The '3-6-9 rule' is useful to remember the upper limit of the normal diameter in centimetres of the small bowel, large bowel and the caecum, respectively. The distinction between small and large bowel loops can be made by assessing the following features:

Valvulae conniventes vs haustra: Valvulae conniventes are the mucosal folds of the small bowel that begin in the duodenum where they are larger, and gradually these get smaller towards the terminal ileum. On imaging these appear as lines that traverse the diameter of the entire lumen of the small bowel (see Figures 2.1 and 2.4a). Large bowel loops can be determined by the presence of haustra, which are the mucosal folds of the colon, and do not traverse the entire length of the lumen on imaging (see Figure 2.4b).

Central location: the small bowel is usually located centrally on imaging compared to large bowel, which runs in the periphery of the abdomen (compare Figures 2.4a and 2.4b).

Absence of faeces: It is unusual for the small bowel to contain formed stool, which has a mottled appearance. The presence of faeces within the bowel lumen suggests it is more likely to be the large bowel.

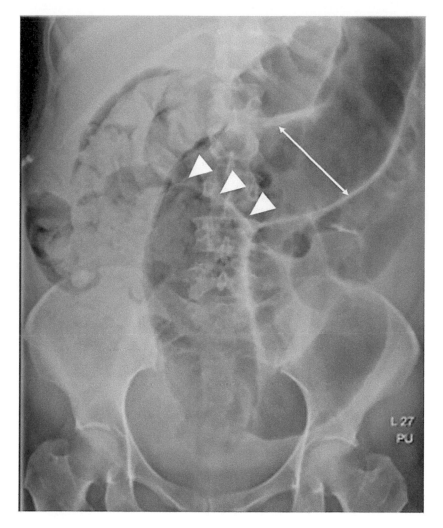

Figure 2.1 AXR showing small bowel obstruction indicated by the dilated small bowel loops. Arrowheads show the valvulae conniventes, which traverse the diameter of the small bowel loop. The double-headed arrow shows the diameter of a dilated loop of small bowel, measuring greater than 3 cm in cases of small bowel obstruction.

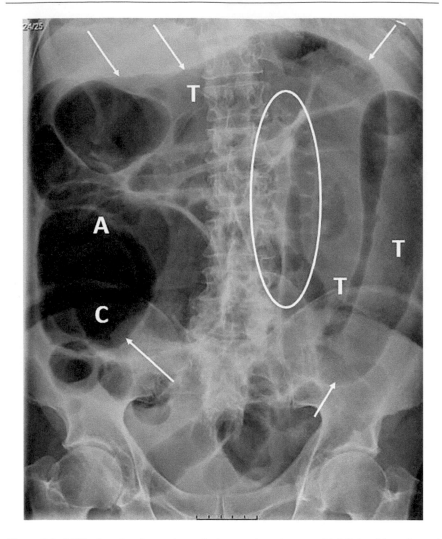

Figure 2.2 AXR showing large bowel obstruction. Arrows highlight dilatation of
the majority of the large bowel, from the caecum (C), through to the
ascending colon (A) and the transverse colon (T). Note the centrally
located dilated loop of the small bowel (marked by the oval), indicates
the ileocaecal valve is incompetent.

Occasionally, the bowel loops may be completely fluid filled, and this can
give the deceiving appearance of a 'gasless' abdomen where there are no
apparent bowel loops on X-ray. CT scan is the imaging of choice if there
is ongoing clinical suspicion in the context of an unremarkable abdominal
radiograph.

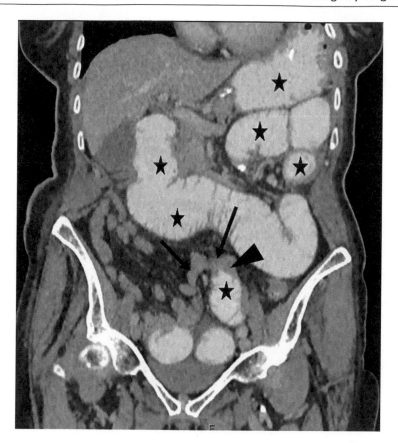

Figure 2.3 Coronal CT showing small bowel obstruction (SBO). The patient has been given oral contrast, which highlights the dilated loops of the small bowel (indicated with the stars). The arrowhead highlights the sharp change in calibre at the level of adhesions known as the transition point of the small bowel from dilated to collapsed small bowel loops. The arrows highlight the efferent collapsed loops distal to the obstruction.

CT

On CT, a mechanical obstruction shows a sharp change in calibre from dilated to collapsed loops at the fulcrum known as the 'transition point', which corresponds to the site of the obstruction (Figure 2.3). Paralytic ileus is characterised by the presence of dilated small bowel with no sharp transition point, rather the calibre of the bowel loops typically smoothly tapers in size. In pseudo-obstruction, typically the large bowel loops are dilated through to the rectum. When assessing these scans, the radiologist/surgeon needs to follow the bowel loops in their entirety by scrolling up and down through the axial images. Due to the length of bowel loops, and in particular the small bowel, it is easy to lose track of which loop of bowel is being examined, especially if they lie on top of one another. In this case, although it can be time consuming, it is important to start again to confidently ensure the whole length of bowel has been examined.

Small Bowel Obstruction

Small bowel obstruction (SBO) is a common cause of emergency admissions and presents classically with vomiting, abdominal pain, abdominal distension and absolute constipation. The most common cause of small bowel obstruction in the West is adhesions in patients who have had previous surgery, followed by hernias. Imaging plays a critical role, particularly in the management of adhesional small bowel obstruction. Occasionally, in the context of a patient presenting with small bowel obstruction, the CT may be reported as showing a closed loop obstruction independent of the ileocaecal valve. This suggests the presence of two transition points in the small bowel with dilated small bowel in between. This may for instance be caused by an internal hernia or adhesions at two points. In patients with a closed loop obstruction, urgent surgical exploration is usually required to prevent ischaemia and perforation.

The cause of small bowel obstruction in patients with a history of abdominal surgery is usually adhesional, and first-line treatment in uncomplicated cases is usually conservative. After clinical assessment and usually an AXR, the first presentation should be confirmed with CT abdomen and pelvis. Gastrograffin, a water-soluble contrast, is given intravenously as a standard, but it can also be given orally to these patients at the time of CT. It is an investigative tool used to highlight the loops of the bowel and therefore potentially the transition point, which can guide management. Gastrograffin can be given orally or via the nasogastric (NG) tube as a 100 mL bolus. If not given at the time of CT, it can be given afterwards once the diagnosis has been confirmed. Following administration, an abdominal radiograph is carried out at least four to six hours later to assess passage of the contrast through the bowel and can be repeated up to 24 hours after. Gastrograffin used in this way is utilised to predict which patients will respond to conservative treatment (3). It has also been shown to reduce the length of hospital stay for these patients (4). The presence of gastrograffin in the colon suggests that the obstruction is not complete and is a good predictor of the success of conservative treatment (Figure 2.4a,b).

Small bowel obstruction caused by hernias is covered in the section below on 'Strangulated Hernia'.

Large Bowel Obstruction

The most common causes of large bowel obstruction are malignancy (60%), diverticular stricture (20%) and sigmoid volvulus (5%). Plain abdominal X-ray can be used to diagnose the presence of large bowel obstruction (Figure 2.2). In large bowel obstruction, both the small bowel and large bowel are usually dilated (the large bowel diameter should normally be less than

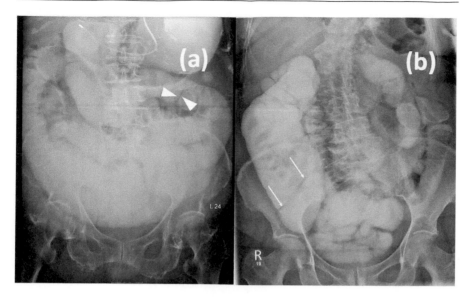

Figure 2.4 Gastrograffin follow-through studies.

(a) Gastrograffin in the dilated small bowel. Note the centrally located loops and the valvulae conniventes (arrowheads highlighting one).

(b) Gastrograffin in the right colon in a different patient, note the right-sided peripheral location of the bowel loop and the haustra (arrows), which do not traverse the full diameter of the bowel loop. Presence of gastrograffin in the colon on the delayed film predicts likely resolution of small bowel obstruction with conservative treatment. Usually, this coincides with the patient opening their bowels.

6 cm), unless there is a closed loop obstruction due to a competent ileocaecal valve, in which case the small bowel will be of normal calibre. In closed loop obstruction, the large bowel cannot decompress into the proximal loops, leading to progressive distension of the large bowel, with a resultant risk of ischaemia and perforation. The caecum is the most vulnerable part of the colon for this complication to occur (Figure 2.5). While a CT scan may show the cause of large bowel obstruction, for example, a stricturing lesion in the large bowel at the point of obstruction as shown in Figure 2.6, it can be difficult to determine the cause on CT imaging alone. The diagnosis usually needs to be confirmed either by direct visualisation using flexisigmoidoscopy or histologically after resection to determine whether a benign or malignant stricture is present.

Sigmoid Volvulus

It is important to differentiate sigmoid volvulus from other causes of large bowel obstruction as the management is usually non-surgical. Abdominal

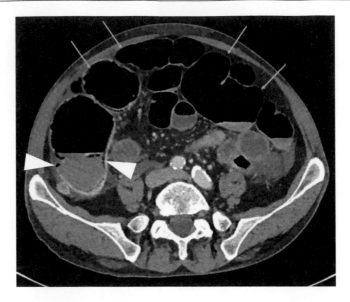

Figure 2.5 Axial contrast-enhanced CT through the abdomen. Arrows show peripherally located dilated loops of the large bowel. Arrowhead showing intramural gas is indicative of ischaemia, a complication of large bowel obstruction.

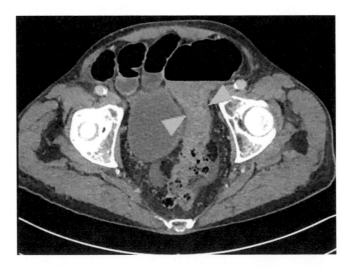

Figure 2.6 Axial contrast-enhanced CT through the abdomen. Arrowheads show diffuse mural thickening of the sigmoid colon, on a background of sigmoid diverticulosis; therefore, the likely cause of the large bowel obstruction in this case is a sigmoid diverticular stricture, but a sigmoid malignancy is also possible, and the cause needs to be confirmed with colonoscopy and biopsy or histologically after surgery.

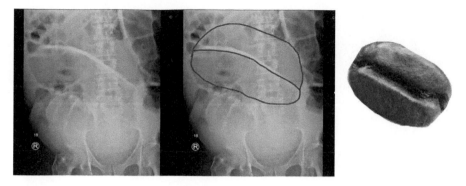

Figure 2.7 AXR showing the 'coffee bean sign' in a case of sigmoid volvulus.

radiographs typically show a 'coffee bean' sign due to a distended sigmoid colon, with the mesenteric axis seen as a thick, white line extending from the right upper quadrant to the left iliac fossa (Figure 2.7).

ACUTE APPENDICITIS

US

Transabdominal US is a useful first-line investigation in females or children presenting with right iliac fossa pain. It is readily available, does not use ionising radiation and does not require any preparation. However, the presence of overlying bowel gas or failure to visualise the appendix may lead to false negatives. US is also operator dependent. On US, the appendix may be seen as a blind-ended tubular structure arising from the caecal pole that does not demonstrate peristalsis (Figure 2.8a). The normal appendix has a diameter of less than 6 mm and is usually compressible without pain with the ultrasound probe. An inflamed appendix typically has a diameter greater than 6 mm. The walls of the inflamed appendix are hypoechoic and usually thicker than 2 mm. The concentric layers of the appendix may be lost, particularly in gangrenous appendicitis, and a hyperechoic appendicolith may be detected at the appendix base. There may be a hyperechoic reaction in the adjacent mesenteric fat in keeping with inflammation. Perforation of the appendix may be detected as discontinuity of the appendix wall. An adjacent abscess or collection may also be detected. While US cannot always visualise the appendix, secondary features of appendicitis may be visible, such as the presence of free fluid. It is also useful to identify other causes, such as mesenteric adenitis in children. Under Doppler, an inflamed appendix may show increased vascularity. In addition to transabdominal ultrasound, transvaginal ultrasound (TVUS) is useful in women of reproductive age as it can exclude other causes of abdominal pain such as

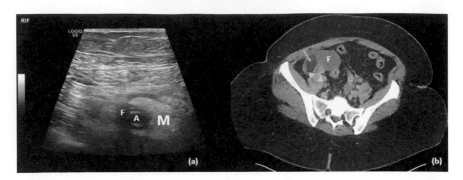

Figure 2.8 (a) Transabdominal US showing a dilated appendix (A) surrounded by periappendiceal fluid (F) and an inflamed mesentry (M). (b) Axial CT of the same patient showing an inflamed appendix, which has an increased diameter indicated by the arrowheads. (F) denotes the same periappendiceal collection as seen in (a), is in keeping with an abscess, secondary to a contained perforation. The arrow shows periappendiceal fat stranding secondary to the inflammation.

gynaecological pathology, including ovarian cysts and pelvic inflammatory disease.

CT

CT is more sensitive than US, but the diagnostic criteria remain largely the same. A diameter of 6 mm or more of the appendix and wall thickness of 2 mm or more with peri-appendicular fat stranding suggests inflammation of the appendix (Figure 2.8b). A calcified appendicolith may also be present.

The presence of an abscess adjacent to the appendix suggests a contained perforation. Contrast CT and examination of the portal venous phase shows ring-shaped enhancement of the wall of the appendix, which is highly suggestive for appendicitis. Contrast also helps define abscesses by enhancing their walls. The sensitivity and specificity of CT scan in the diagnosis of appendicitis is 91% and 90%, respectively. Another advantage of CT is in the diagnosis of alternative causes of abdominal pain, for example:

- Mesenteric lymphadenitis
- Caecal carcinoma
- Epiploic appendagitis
- Cystitis
- Urolithiasis
- Tubo-ovarian abscess
- Ovarian cyst torsion

Low-dose unenhanced CT yields equivalent sensitivity and specificity to standard CT with contrast and is a useful protocol in younger patients.

Appendicitis in Pregnancy

As CT is contraindicated in pregnant women; US and non-contrast MRI (contrast-enhanced MRI is contraindicated in pregnancy) are alternative available imaging modalities, depending on the stage of pregnancy, as the appendix is less well visualised on US with increasing gestation, and MRI is not usually performed in the first trimester. MRI can provide excellent views of the appendix, and sensitivity and specificity are between 90% and 100%.

Appendicitis in Children

US is the first-line imaging modality for suspected appendicitis in children. It can be difficult to visualise the appendix on US, for example, in the case of a retrocaecal appendix that will be obscured by bowel gas. In these cases, secondary features such as free fluid may indicate appendicitis or a perforated appendix. If there is diagnostic uncertainty after US, CT may be required for confirmation. US can also be useful to exclude appendicitis where there is clinical uncertainty by looking for alternative causes of pain, such as enlarged mesenteric lymph nodes in mesenteric adenitis. In older females, US can be used to look for gynaecological causes of pain. US is also useful for confirming the diagnosis of an appendix mass in young children. In this case where conservative treatment is undertaken, US can be used to guide drainage of any collections. US may then also be used for monitoring those patients having conservative treatment.

STRANGULATED HERNIA

Uncomplicated abdominal hernias are commonly visualised on imaging incidentally, where they can contain intraabdominal fat and non-dilated loops of bowel. An obstructed hernia can be confirmed on imaging, usually CT (see Figure 2.9a,b), and in these cases the transition point is at the level of the hernia neck. Evidence of strangulation of fat or the small bowel may be seen as fat stranding or adjacent fluid or oedema.

INTUSSUSCEPTION

Intussusception is another cause of mechanical bowel obstruction that is diagnosed on imaging. The appearances on imaging are quite specific, whereby the proximal portion of bowel, often with some of its fatty mesentery, interposes into the lumen of the immediate distal portion. This results in a 'pseudokidney sign' due to the reniform shape of the intussusception and the central mesenteric fat that imitates perinephric fat (Figure 2.10). Dilated bowel loops are seen proximal to the intussusception due to the obstruction that ensues. It is important to establish on imaging whether there is

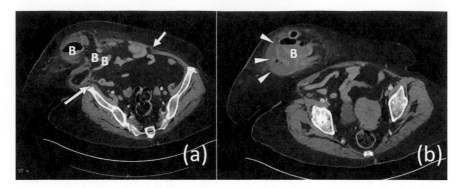

Figure 2.9 (a) Contrast-enhanced axial CT of the abdomen. The arrows define the width of the hernia neck. The hernia contains loops of the small bowel (B) and stranding in the surrounding subcutaneous abdominal fat. (b) Contrast-enhanced axial CT of the abdomen. The hernia contains dilated small bowel loops and free fluid (arrowheads) due to obstruction caused by the hernia.

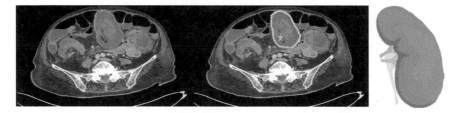

Figure 2.10 Contrast-enhanced axial CT scan. The outline shows the reniform shape of the intussusception. The star highlights the mesenteric fat trapped inside the interposed bowel loops, which is reminiscent of perinephric fat.

any structural cause, for example, a malignancy acting as lead point for the intussusception. In the case of malignancy, the lesion may be obscured and hidden amongst the interposed loops of the bowel; in this case, looking for secondary features such as pathological mesenteric and retroperitoneal nodes is important.

BOERHAAVE'S SYNDROME

Boerhaave's syndrome is a condition characterised by oesophageal rupture. This usually occurs after excessive vomiting. CT chest may show pneumo-mediastinum due to the presence of air leak from the site of perforation. However, the presence of pneumomediastinum alone does not confirm an oesophageal perforation. As per other sites of perforation, looking at the

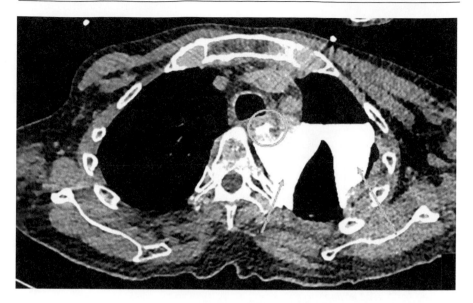

Figure 2.11 Axial CT chest with oral contrast. The contrast-filled oesophagus is highlighted by a circle. The oesophageal perforation has given rise to a fistula with the left pleural cavity, resulting in the passage of oral contrast into it (arrow).

images on lung windows is important to better highlight the presence of air. It is worth noting that pneumomediastinum may also be caused by pneumothorax due to excessive pressure on the airways caused by vomiting. In this case repeating the CT with oral contrast is important to confirm whether there is an oesophageal perforation or not.

CT chest and abdomen performed after administering oral water-soluble contrast is used to identify the presence of a perforation; the oral contrast can highlight the site of the perforation, although the actual mural defect is often difficult to see. Secondary features such as a pleural effusion containing contrast may clinch the diagnosis and is seen due to the pleuro-oesophageal fistula that has been fashioned by the perforation (Figure 2.11).

ACUTE GASTRIC DILATATION/GASTRIC OUTLET OBSTRUCTION

Acute gastric dilatation may occur due to non-mechanical causes such as gastroparesis seen more commonly in diabetics or due to a mechanical obstruction of the gastric outflow tract by a lesion such as lymphoma. It may require urgent decompression with an NG tube to prevent gastric ischaemia and perforation. This condition can be diagnosed on CT and sometimes the cause may also be seen; however, an endoscopy is often required to establish the aetiology.

ACUTE GASTROINTESTINAL PERFORATION

Acute GI perforation typically presents with acute abdominal pain and peritonitis. Erect chest radiograph may be sufficient to make a diagnosis in the presence of a consistent history, but CT scan is usually requested to confirm the diagnosis and confirm the cause, though sometimes it is difficult to differentiate an upper GI from lower GI perforation.

X-Ray

A suspected bowel perforation is the only indication for an erect CXR. The key is looking for free gas beneath the right hemidiaphragm. Gas does collect beneath the left hemidiaphragm; however, the stomach gas bubble can obscure and confuse the picture. There is no anatomical gas beneath the right hemidiaphragm, so it is more reliable to scrutinise this site for free gas (Figure 2.12).

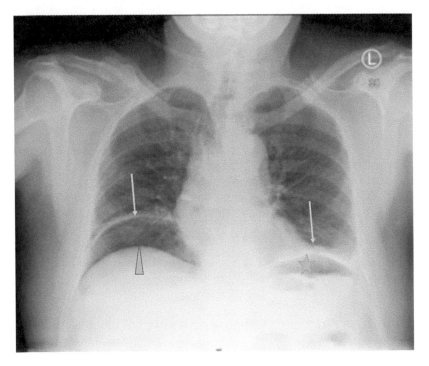

Figure 2.12 Erect chest radiograph. Arrows show the arches of the hemidiaphragms; the arrowhead depicts the free edge of the liver. Between the arrow and the arrowhead, free gas has collected; in the absence of recent abdominal surgery, this is always pathological and indicative of a perforated viscus. Always look for the free gas on the right side in this position as the gas in the stomach bubble on the left (star) can obscure or be confused with free gas.

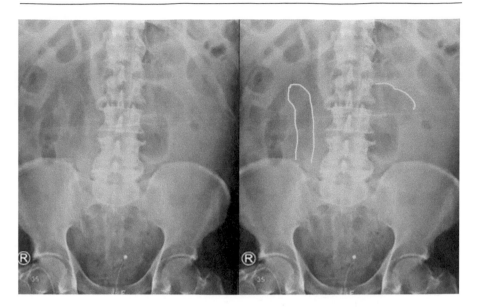

Figure 2.13 AXR showing intraperitoneal free gas is in keeping with bowel perforation. The duplicate image on the right highlights 'non-anatomical gas (NAG)' lying free in the peritoneum, which is not conforming to the shape of a bowel loop. The outlines depict a loop of small bowel. Note that both the inner (epithelial) and outer (serosal) sides of the bowel wall are visible as a white stripe on the image on the left, as gas is present on both sides of the bowel (pathologically on the serosal side), which highlights it.

AXRs are usually performed at the same time as an erect CXR. It can be difficult to spot free gas on the AXR. The key is looking for non-anatomical gas (NAG) lying free in the peritoneal cavity, i.e., gas that is not sited within a bowel lumen. When this occurs, the gas cannot be compartmentalised into either a small or large bowel loop as it highlights structures not usually seen on AXR. When there is a large amount of free air, Rigler's sign may be seen (Figure 2.13), which is the presence of air on both sides of the bowel wall, highlighting the bowel wall on X-ray.

CT

On CT as the patients are lying prone, free gas settles in an ante-dependent position anteriorly in the peritoneal cavity (Figure 2.14), and in this position the gas highlights the falciform ligament. It is also helpful to use the lung windows in these cases, particularly when there is only a small volume of free gas, where distinguishing it from gas in adjacent bowel can be difficult. The site of perforation may not always be seen, but the location of the air and presence of pathology in the GI tract may help indicate the site of perforation.

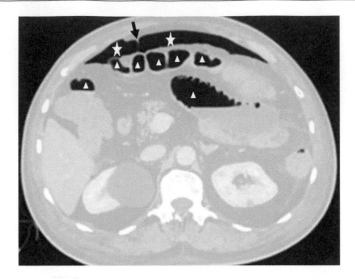

Figure 2.14 Axial CT of the upper abdomen on lung windows. The arrow highlights the falciform ligament. The stars show extraluminal, intraperitoneal gas on either side of the falciform ligament. The arrowheads are contained within intraluminal bowel gas.

GALLSTONE DISEASE

Acute presentations of gallstone disease include biliary colic, acute cholecystitis and obstructive jaundice. The gallbladder, common bile duct (CBD) and gallstones are readily visible in most patients on US, and this is the best modality to assess for gallstone disease (Figure 2.15). In acute cholecystitis, the gallbladder is thick-walled (normal thickness is <3 mm), the gallbladder contents can look hyperechoic and complex, gallstones are often present and there can be fluid surrounding the gallbladder (pericholecystic fluid). In severe cases, the adjacent liver parenchyma can appear heterogeneous, due to secondary hepatic inflammation. A useful sign is the 'sonographic Murphy's sign', whereby the US operator can localise the gallbladder and press on it lightly with the probe, which elicits tenderness in cases of acute cholecystitis.

CT is not the best modality for assessing the gallbladder and for cholelithiasis, but in patients presenting with acute abdominal pain it is often the best modality when imaging is required out of hours or if US is technically difficult, for example, in obese patients (Figure 2.16). It is also useful to exclude other causes of biliary symptoms such as pancreatic malignancy, for example, in patients presenting with obstructive jaundice, and can also detect intra- and extrahepatic duct dilatation. However, stones that are radiolucent will not be apparent on CT, and magnetic resonance cholangiopancreatography (MRCP) may be used in cases where the cause of CBD

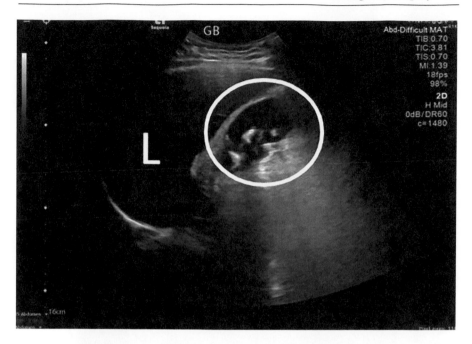

Figure 2.15 Transabdominal US image of the liver (L) and gallbladder. The gallbladder is highlighted with an oval outline. Note the multiple bright
(hyperechoic) foci within the gallbladder representing gallstones.

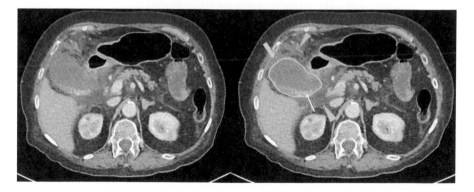

Figure 2.16 Contrast-enhanced axial CT through the upper abdomen, duplicated
and labelled on the right. The outline depicts the wall of the inflamed
gallbladder, which can be difficult to delineate if there is a lot of
pericholecystic fluid (block arrow) and pericholecystic stranding
(arrowhead). The narrower arrow shows multiple small gallstones
layering dependently in the gallbladder.

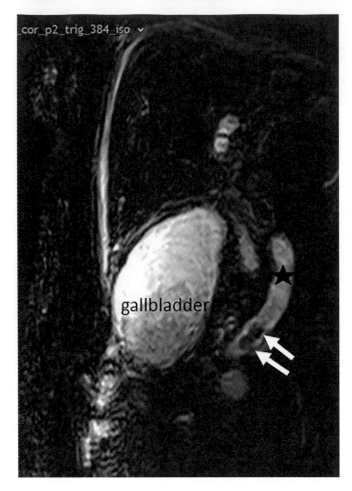

Figure 2.17 MRCP showing filling defects is in keeping with gallstones (arrows) in the dilated CBD (star).

dilatation is not apparent on CT or US. MRCP utilises a sequence that highlights the fluid in the biliary system, thus highlighting any intrinsic biliary filling defects such as gallstones (Figure 2.17).

Intraoperative Cholangiogram

Intraoperative cholangiogram is utilised alongside cholecystectomy to assess the biliary anatomy and to look for bile duct stones intraoperatively (Figure 2.18). It may be used in the emergency setting during hot cholecystectomy as an alternative to MRCP in patients presenting with obstructive jaundice secondary to gallstones. It is also used to visualise the common bile duct to exclude choledocholithiasis in those patients presenting with

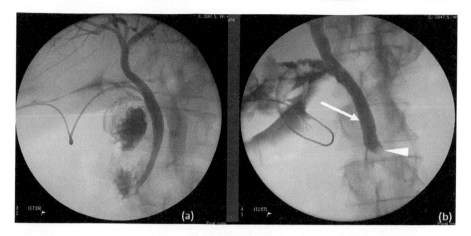

Figure 2.18 Intraoperative cholangiogram. This shows contrast enhancing the biliary and tree and duodenum. (a) On the left, the common bile duct is normal and the left and right hepatic ducts are visible. (b) On the right, the common bile duct is dilated and there is a rounded filling defect in the distal common bile duct (arrow) consistent with a stone (arrowhead).

gallstone pancreatitis, again as an alternative to MRCP. For anatomy, in rare cases the cystic duct drains directly into the right hepatic duct, where it has a higher chance of injury. It is important to visualise proximal filling of the hepatic ducts and see the left and right hepatic duct bifurcation to make sure that no bile duct injury has occurred.

ACUTE PANCREATITIS

For assessment of pancreatitis and its complications, CT is used; however, in mild pancreatitis, the CT scan may be normal. Necrosis develops a few days after onset; therefore, CT is usually not useful in the first few days unless there is diagnostic uncertainty in patients presenting with acute abdominal pain or in patients presenting clinically with severe pancreatitis. CT findings in acute pancreatitis include a swollen oedematous pancreas (5) and peri-pancreatic fat stranding (Figure 2.19a). Radio-opaque gallstones may be seen in the biliary tree in gallstone-induced pancreatitis as well as any associated duct dilatation. Complications include splenic vein thrombosis, splenic artery pseudoaneurysm, necrosis (Figure 2.19b), large collection and eventually pseudocyst (Figure 2.19c). Serial CT scans are particularly important in assessing evolution of complications of pancreatitis in patients with severe disease. For example, necrosis may develop into a collection or pseudocyst that may require future drainage.

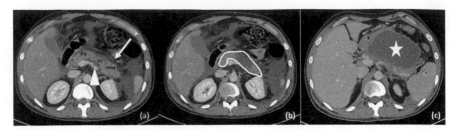

Figure 2.19 Complications of acute pancreatitis. (a) Contrast-enhanced axial
CT through the upper abdomen in a case of acute pancreatitis. The
pancreas is swollen secondary to inflammatory oedema. The fat surrounding the pancreas contains stranding due to the inflammation
(arrow). Note the filling defect in the splenic vein (arrowhead) in
keeping with thrombosis. (b) The outline of the pancreas is highlighted on this contrast-enhanced CT. Note the lack of enhancement
in the body of the pancreas is in keeping with necrosis. (c) The star
highlights a pancreatic pseudocyst that has arisen as a late complication of pancreatitis.

CHRONIC PANCREATITIS

Characteristics of chronic pancreatitis on CT include punctate small foci
of calcification distributed throughout the pancreas, which is usually
atrophic. It is also important to look at the location of any pancreatic stones
(Figure 2.20) as intraductal stones may cause obstruction of the pancreatic
duct and may need intervention to reduce pain and prevent further episodes
of pancreatitis as opposed to parenchymal stones.

DIVERTICULAR DISEASE

Diverticular disease is characterised according to the modified Hinchey classification, which describes six stages or complications of the disease. CT is
used to stratify the disease and aids in deciding the appropriate management
(Table 2.1).

Stage 0 and 1A disease can be managed conservatively with antibiotics.
If a localised abscess is seen on CT, particularly those greater than 3 cm
in diameter, it may be amenable to drainage under CT or US guidance, to
reduce sepsis and expedite recovery (Figure 2.21). As they are contained and
contain fluid and gas, pericolic collections can be mistaken on CT for normal loops of adjacent bowel so it is important to ensure that what is felt to
be a bowel loop does communicate anatomically with adjacent loops of the
bowel via their lumens. The presence of generalised pus or faeculant peritonitis usually requires a laparotomy. Sometimes the CT scan shows generalised
free air or fluid but the source of perforation is not clear and can only be

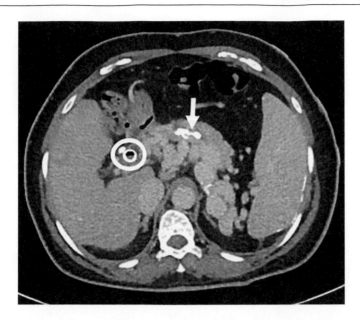

Figure 2.20 Contrast-enhanced axial CT showing intraductal pancreatic calculi (marked by arrow) on a background of an atrophied, chronically inflamed pancreas. Note the CBD stent highlighted with a circle.

Table 2.1 Severity Stratification of Acute Diverticulitis According to CT Scan Findings

Stage	Clinical	CT Findings
0	Mild clinical diverticulitis	Diverticula with colonic wall thickening
1A	Confined pericolic inflammation or phlegmon	Pericolic soft tissue changes
1B	Pericolic or mesocolic abscess	1A changes and pericolic or mesocolic abscess
2	Pelvic, distant intra-abdominal or retroperitoneal abscess	Distant abscess
3	Generalised purulent peritonitis	Localised or generalised ascites, pneumoperitoneum, peritoneal thickening
4	Generalised faecal peritonitis	Same as stage 3

confirmed at the time of laparotomy; however, looking for evidence of acute diverticulitis on the scan can help direct the surgeon to this being the likely cause. Patients who are treated conservatively should be followed up with a flexible sigmoidoscopy or colonoscopy after six weeks, once the episode has subsided to exclude a colonic malignancy, which may be missed on CT due to the acute inflammation masking it.

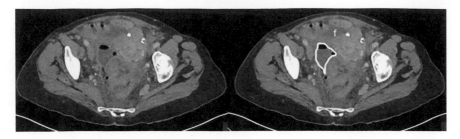

Figure 2.21 Axial CT of the pelvis. The duplicate image on the right contains the label. The outline of a diverticular abscess is shown on the image on the right. Note the diffuse fat stranding in the pelvic fat and the presence of free fluid (f).

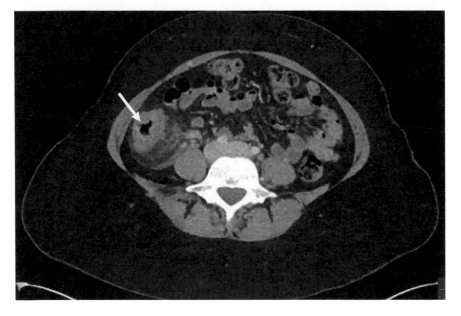

Figure 2.22 Contrast-enhanced axial CT. The arrow labels diffusely thickened ascending colon associated with surrounding mesenteric fat stranding, in keeping with acute colitis.

ACUTE COLITIS

Acute colitis manifests as diffuse thickening of the bowel wall on CT scan (Figure 2.22). There may be associated surrounding mesenteric fat stranding and free fluid. US can be helpful, especially in thinner and younger patients, and may show thickened bowel wall and increased blood flow on Doppler.

Various causes of the colitis should be considered when scrutinising the scan, including:

- *Inflammatory bowel disease*: Look for other features such as contiguous large bowel loop involvement in ulcerative colitis and skip lesions and terminal ileitis in Crohn's disease.
- *Ischaemic colitis*: Scrutinise the mesenteric arteries and coeliac axis for any focal critical narrowing or for the presence of a vascular filling defect (especially in patients with predisposing conditions such as atrial fibrillation and endocarditis). The mucosa may not enhance as well with contrast and, anatomically, the portions of bowel involved may follow a vascular territory pattern.
- *Infective colitis*: Non-specific distribution of colitis often with a clinical history of infective symptoms.

ACUTE GYNAECOLOGICAL DISEASE

Gynaecological disease is usually considered as a differential diagnosis, along with acute appendicitis in female patients presenting with right iliac fossa pain (Figure 2.23). Tubo-ovarian abscesses are a source of sepsis and can mimic acute appendicitis both clinically and sometimes radiological differentiation is also difficult. Transvaginal ultrasound scan is the best modality to assess the female pelvis for gynaecological conditions. Transabdominal pelvic US is a useful alternative in patients who have never been sexually active, particularly if they are slim. In the case of transabdominal pelvic US, it is helpful to instruct the patient to have a full bladder, as this forms a useful window to inspect the pelvic organs. While CT scan may show an abscess, sometimes it is difficult to differentiate a tubo-ovarian abscess from an appendicular abscess, particularly in patients with little mesenteric fat and therefore less clear definition on the anatomical planes on CT. On the left side it can be difficult to differentiate a tubo-ovarian abscess from a diverticular abscess on CT scan. In these cases, the combination of CT scan and ultrasound provides the most useful information.

GASTROINTESTINAL BLEEDING

Gastrointestinal bleeding is traditionally characterised into two types. Bleeding proximal to the ligament of Treitz is defined as an upper GI bleed as opposed to bleeding distal to the ligament of Treitz, which is referred to as a lower GI bleed. CT angiogram is useful in the acute setting, but it is only sensitive if the patient is actively bleeding, with some studies quoting a minimum rate of 0.25 mLs/min (6). CT angiogram not only identifies the site of bleeding (Figure 2.24a,b) but it may also identify any pathological

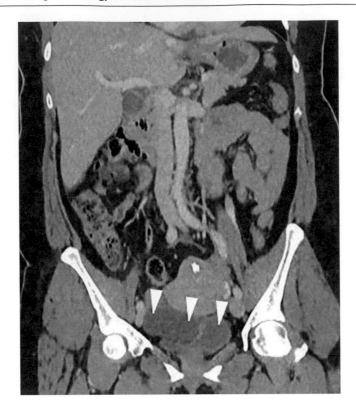

Figure 2.23 Coronal contrast-enhanced CT showing a dilated, fluid-filled, right-sided fallopian tube highlighted with the arrowheads; in the context of pelvic sepsis, this was diagnosed as a tubo-ovarian abscess.

cause. If a terminal cause is established, then this may guide ceilings of care in an unwell patient.

It can also help plan further radiological intervention, in particular fluoroscopic angiography and embolisation. CT angiogram is performed after administering iodinated intravenous contrast. A non-contrast phase is initially performed (7). This phase is useful to look for highly attenuating objects that may mimic pathology or acute haemorrhage on a contrast CT scan such as calcified material, opaque foreign bodies, clips or luminal contrast material. It may also show recent unclotted/layering of intraluminal blood to help localise the source of a bleed. Arterial and portal venous phases are then taken. In the case of active arterial bleeding, the arterial phase can show intraluminal extravasion of dense contrast (Figure 2.24a). In addition, the arterial anatomy and any anomalies such as arteriovenous malformations or highly vascular tumours such as carcinoids can be highlighted during this phase. Due to the dynamic nature of this study with scans acquired at different time points after the administration of intravenous

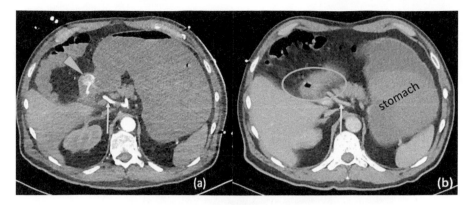

Figure 2.24 (a) Arterial phase of a triple-phase CT angiogram. The arrow high-lights the normal bright arterial enhancement of the left gastric artery after it has arisen from the coeliac trunk (not shown). The arrowhead highlights the disorganised extraluminal pathological enhancement of active arterial extravasation of contrast at the level of the pylorus. (b) Delayed (portal venous phase) of a CT angiogram in the same patient. The oval at the same site of the active arterial bleed in (a) shows the dispersal of the bright contrast from the arterial extravasation. Note the layering of different density material is in keeping with clotted blood and contrast that fills the stomach. Urgent interventional radiology input is required in this case.

contrast, an active arterial bleed that appears as extravasation on the arterial phase study usually alters in its configuration on the delayed portal venous phase (Figure 2.24b), and this observation aids in the detection of an active haemorrhage. The delayed portal venous phase is also used to assess for any associated or causative pathology such as malignancy. Although CT angiogram is less sensitive for detecting lower-flow bleeds, a negative CT angiogram is also useful as these patients are less likely to need intervention to control the bleeding and can usually be observed.

PERIANAL SEPSIS

The term 'perianal sepsis' refers to perianal abscesses, ischiorectal abscesses and fistula-in-ano. Most cases of perianal and ischiorectal abscesses do not require imaging. A clinical assessment should be carried out, and if appropriate they can be managed with incision and drainage. CT can identify perianal sepsis in patients being investigated for sepsis of unknown cause. Perianal fistulas are covered in the Colorectal Surgery chapter.

Perianal abscesses on CT give the appearance of a collection of fluid, which may contain air. Sometimes the wall is thickened and there may be surrounding inflammation. CT can provide information regarding the

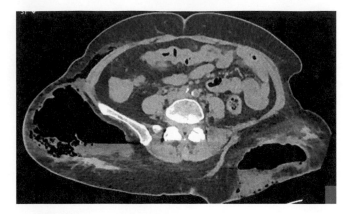

Figure 2.25 Axial CT through the abdomen showing dissection of gas from perianal sepsis that has extended into the subcutaneous plane of the
lower back and right anterior abdomen with extension to the skin
surface on the left side. Necrotising fasciitis is a consideration in
this patient.

location and extent of any abscesses. In the presence of air in the soft tissues,
the diagnosis of necrotising fasciitis must also be considered (Figure 2.25).
In these cases, CT scan can help map the involvement of the tissues prior to
surgical debridement.

ABDOMINAL TRAUMA

Abdominal trauma affecting solid abdominal viscera is mostly assessed by
trauma CT as part of a dedicated trauma protocol. Intravenous contrast will
usually be administered to detect active extravasation (i.e. bleeding) that
may require urgent attention by an interventional radiologist.

Pancreatic Trauma

Pancreatic trauma is uncommon, occurring in around 4% of patients with
abdominal injuries. Isolated injury to the pancreas is rare, as it is intimately
related to several vital structures including the duodenum, spleen and major
vessels such as the superior mesenteric vessels and splenic vessels. Damage
to the main pancreatic duct occurs in 15% of cases and is a cause of major
morbidity and mortality due to the corrosive nature of pancreatic juice on
nearby structures.

A grading system for the severity of injury is provided by the American
Association for the Surgery of Trauma (Figure 2.26).

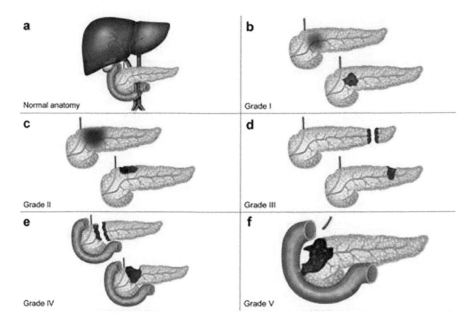

Figure 2.26 Grading the severity of pancreatic injury: grade I – minor contusion or laceration with no duct injury, grade II – major contusion or laceration with no duct injury, grade III – transection or major laceration with duct disruption in distal pancreas, grade IV – transection of proximal pancreas or major laceration with associated injury to the ampulla, grade V – massive disruption of the pancreatic head. Taken with permission from (8).

CT is the imaging modality of choice, and patients are often assessed on imaging as part of the major trauma protocol. It can be difficult to accurately grade the pancreatic injury on CT due to the pro-inflammatory effect of the leaking pancreatic juices.

Splenic Trauma

The American Association for the Surgery of Trauma (AAST) has published the most widely used grading system for splenic injuries and is based on the CT findings (Table 2.2); the injuries are often assessed on CT as part of the major trauma protocol (Figure 2.27).

Treatment of splenic injuries tends to be non-operative, which has a failure rate of around 10%. Preservation of the spleen is important to reduce the risk of Overwhelming Post-Splenectomy Infection Syndrome (OPSI).

Table 2.2 The American Association for the Surgery of Trauma (AAST) Grading
System for Splenic Injuries Based on CT Findings

Grade	Imaging Criteria (CT Findings)
I	Subcapsular haematoma <10% surface area
	Parenchymal laceration <1 cm depth
	Capsular tear
II	Subcapsular haematoma 10–50% surface area; intraparenchymal haematoma <5 cm
	Parenchymal laceration 1–3 cm
III	Subcapsular haematoma >50% surface area; ruptured subcapsular or intraparenchymal haematoma ≥5 cm
	Parenchymal laceration >3 cm depth
IV	Any injury in the presence of a splenic vascular injury or active bleeding confined within splenic capsule
	Parenchymal laceration involving segmental or hilar vessels producing >25% devascularisation
V	Any injury in the presence of a splenic vascular injury with active bleeding extended beyond the spleen into the peritoneum
	Shattered spleen

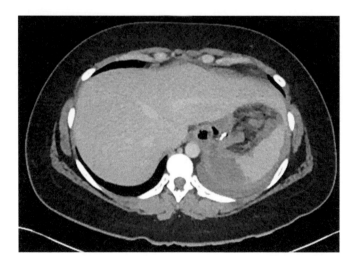

Figure 2.27 Axial CT through the upper abdomen showing a grade II laceration
of the spleen.

Liver Trauma

The American Association for the Surgery of Trauma grading classification
is as follows; once again, this is based on the CT findings (Table 2.3). The
injuries are often assessed on CT as part of the major trauma protocol.

Table 2.3 The American Association for the Surgery of Trauma (AAST) Grading System for Liver Injuries Based on CT Findings

Grade	CT Findings
I	Subcapsular haematoma <10% surface area Parenchymal laceration <1 cm length
II	Subcapsular haematoma 10–15% surface area Intraparenchymal haematoma <10 cm diameter Laceration 1–3 cm in depth and ≤10 cm length
III	Subcapsular haematoma >50% surface area; ruptured subcapsular or parenchymal haematoma Intraparenchymal laceration >10 cm Laceration >3 cm depth Any injury in the presence of a liver vascular injury or active bleeding contained within liver parenchyma
IV	Parenchymal disruption involving 25–75% of a hepatic lobe Active bleeding extending beyond the liver parenchyma into the peritoneum
V	Parenchymal disruption >75% of hepatic lobe Juxtahepatic venous injury to include retrohepatic vena cava and central major hepatic veins

If more than two grades of injury are present, the higher grade of injury is used.

Vascular injury is defined as a pseudoaneurysm or arteriovenous fistula and appears as a focal collection of vascular contrast that decreases in attenuation with delayed imaging. Active bleeding from a vascular injury presents as vascular contrast, focal or diffuse, which increases in size or attenuation in delayed phase. Vascular thrombosis can lead to organ infarction. If there is more than one injury, one grade point is added up to grade III.

REFERENCES

1. Association of Surgeons of Great Britain and Ireland and the Royal College of Surgeons of England. Commissioning Guide: Emergency General Surgery (Acute Abdominal Pain) 2014.
2. Nelms David W et al. Clin Colon Rectal Surg (2021). PMC8292005
3. Abbas S et al. Cochrane Database Syst. Rev. (2007). PMC6465054
4. Ceresoli M et al. Am J Surg. (2016). PMID: 26329902
5. Koo BC et al. Br J Radiol. (2010). PMCID: PMC3473535.
6. Dobritz M et al. Eur Radiol. (2009). PMID: 19588146
7. Wells M et al. Radiographics. (2018). PMID: 29883267.
8. Søreide K, Weiser TG, Parks RW. Clinical update on management of pancreatic trauma. HPB (Oxford). 2018 Dec;20(12):1099–1108. doi: 10.1016/j.hpb.2018.05.009. Epub 2018 Jul 11. PMID: 30005994.

Chapter 3

Upper GI and HPB

THE OESOPHAGUS

Radiological assessment of the oesophagus is usually done after or in conjunction with direct visualisation with UGI endoscopy. Generally, in cases of benign disease, the oesophagus is usually radiologically assessed fluoroscopically by barium swallow. CT and PET-CT can also be utilised to assess for malignancy. Conventional transcutaneous US can assess the cervical portion of the oesophagus, but the majority of the oesophagus as it descends into the chest cannot be imaged in this way; rather, if there is concern regarding malignancy, endoscopic ultrasound (EUS) can be used.

Gastro-Oesophageal Reflux Disease (GORD)

GORD can result in a number of symptoms, including heartburn and dysphagia. A barium swallow is a test that is performed under fluoroscopic guidance, whereby a barium bolus (barium is exceptionally radiodense) is swallowed and opacifies the lumen of the upper aerodigestive tract and the oesophagus. It is a dynamic study meaning the detail of the swallow and the passage of the bolus through the oesophagus and into the stomach is seen in real time; therefore, any issues with motility and filling defects within the upper aerodigestive tract and oesophagus can be seen. Harnessing the dynamic nature of this study is also useful for assessment of gastro-oesophageal reflux as the contrast bolus can be seen to pass into the stomach and then return retrogradely into the oesophagus if reflux is present; certain positional manoeuvres to provoke reflux can be adopted by the radiologist/radiographer doing the examination to accentuate the condition.

Achalasia

Achalasia is a primary oesophageal motility disorder defined as a failure of the lower oesophageal sphincter to relax, causing a functional obstruction at the gastro-oesophageal junction. This results in a classical tapering of the

 DOI: 10.1201/9781003324362-3

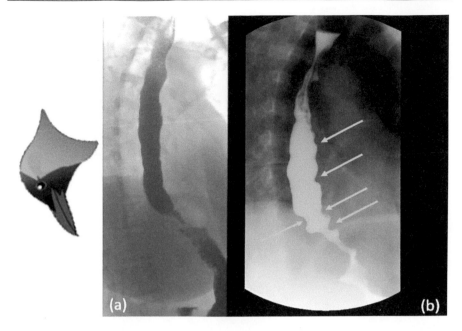

Figure 3.1 (a) Still image from a barium swallow study showing a mildly dilated oesophagus which tapers distally, in keeping with achalasia; note the 'bird's beak' appearance at the distal oesophagus. (b) The indentations of the oesophageal wall (arrows) are known as tertiary contractions, which arise from dysmotility and are often associated with a resultant standing column of contrast in the oesophagus.

distal oesophagus and a 'bird's beak' appearance on barium swallow (see Figure 3.1a), as well as a dilated oesophagus, which often contracts in an uncoordinated way. Other radiological signs can include a small stomach bubble and opacities in the lungs that arise due to aspiration of the contents of the dilated oesophagus.

Motility Disorders

Oesophageal dysmotility is well seen on barium swallow as disorganised, uncoordinated contractions which are non-functional and fail to result in effective peristalsis (Figure 3.1b). These non-functional contractions are known as 'tertiary contractions.' As a result of the oesophageal dysmotility, the passage of contrast through the oesophagus is usually delayed.

Oesophageal Cancer

Imaging plays a key role in staging oesophageal cancer to determine resectability and surgical approach. Initial staging is carried out using CT of the

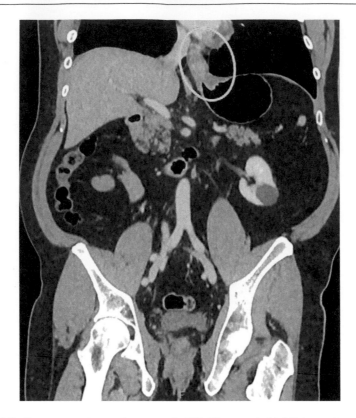

Figure 3.2 Contrast-enhanced coronal CT. The oval highlights circumferential thickening of the distal oesophagus, extending into the gastro-oesophageal junction and on to the fundus of the stomach.

thorax, abdomen and pelvis to assess local extent and to look for metastatic disease (see Figure 3.2). This is particularly important as around 50% of patients have metastatic disease at the time of presentation (1). Local staging of the tumour is then necessary to determine the best treatment approach. Early-stage tumours may be amenable to endoscopic resection. For those tumours that require surgical resection, assessment of the resection margins is important to determine whether local control can be achieved, including craniocaudal and radial margins as well as the presence of lymph node metastases.

Prior to performing a CT scan, distension of the oesophagus is achieved by asking the patient to drink around 200 mL of water. The reformatted images are useful to assess invasion of the tumour into surrounding structures and hence differentiate between T3 and T4 disease. CT is also used for follow-up to assess response to chemotherapy or radiotherapy, and it is also useful in patients with a clinical suspicion of recurrence. In addition, endoscopic ultrasound (EUS) is used for the staging of oesophageal and oesophago-gastric junctional tumours. It provides accurate visualisation of the five layers of the oesophagus and aids the characterisation of the T stage of the tumour; it is also the most accurate imaging modality to assess resectability. For patients with malignant strictures, alternative probes may have to be used, including tapered or mini-probes. The presence of lymph node metastases can also be assessed by EUS with a high sensitivity of around 91%. Four characteristics of the lymph nodes are suggestive, but not diagnostic, of nodal metastatic disease. These include a size above 10 mm, a well-defined boundary, homogeneous low echogenicity and a rounded shape. However, the sensitivity of these findings is quite low and combining EUS and fine needle aspiration (FNA) helps improve the accuracy of diagnosing abnormal lymph nodes.

PET-CT combines anatomical and functional information when assessing a tumour as the majority of oesophageal tumours are FDG (fluorodeoxyglucose) avid. PET-CT can detect tumour and lymph node metastases, and is also useful for detecting distant and occult metastatic disease, as well as detecting suspected residual or recurrent disease not seen on conventional CT.

THE STOMACH

Barium studies traditionally used to assess the stomach have been largely replaced by endoscopy and CT, the latter predominantly used to stage gastric malignancies.

Hiatus Hernia

Hiatus hernias are divided into four types (see Table 3.1).

Table 3.1 Types of Hiatus Hernias

Type	Description
1	This is a sliding hiatus hernia comprising around 95% of cases
2	Paraoesophageal hiatus hernia
3	Mixed-type paraoesophageal hiatus hernia
4	Mixed-type hiatus hernia with additional herniation of viscera

Chest radiograph appearances are characteristic and show a rounded air-fluid level that lies above the diaphragm, often superimposed onto the mediastinum; a typical appearance is shown in Figure 3.3a.

Hiatus hernias are well seen on CT and can often be seen incidentally on CT scan performed for some other purpose (Figure 3.3b).

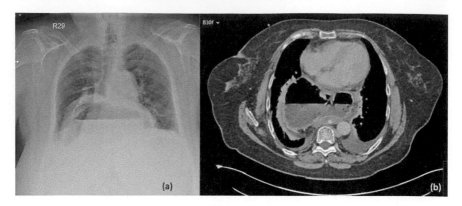

Figure 3.3 (a) Chest radiograph showing a structure with an air-fluid level superimposed onto the mediastinum; the appearances are in keeping with a hiatus hernia. (b) Axial CT of the lower thorax in the same patient as (a) showing the large sliding hiatus hernia in the posterior mediastinum.

Peptic Stricture

Benign peptic stricture may be caused by peptic ulcer disease in the pyloric antrum causing gastric outflow obstruction. This is seen as a dilated stomach on CT scan, which is usually fluid/food filled. With a pyloric stricture, the duodenum is collapsed distal to the stricture.

Gastric Carcinoma

Up to 95% of all gastric malignancies are adenocarcinomas, while the remainder include lymphoma, stromal and neuroendocrine tumours. As with carcinoma of the oesophagus, CT is commonly used for staging of the nodes as well as to determine whether metastatic disease is present. Depending on the size of the malignancy, details about the appearances of the primary tumour may also be rendered from the CT.

Gastrointestinal Stromal Tumours (GISTs)

GISTs are best appreciated at endoscopy but may also be seen on CT. They are the most common mesenchymal tumour of the gastrointestinal tract, and the majority of them occur in the stomach. Around one-quarter of GISTs are malignant. Contrast-enhanced CT is used to radiologically characterise these tumours. The smaller GISTs tend to be solid tumours that can be exophytic (see Figure 3.4) and lie subserosally, intramurally or submucosally; in the case of the latter, the mucosa is usually intact. Larger lesions can appear as a heterogeneously enhancing mass due to internal necrosis, haemorrhage

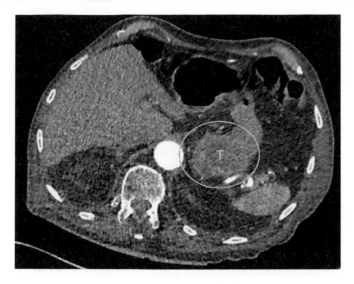

Figure 3.4 Contrast-enhanced axial CT through the upper abdomen showing a poorly enhanced partially exophytic tumour (T) of the stomach highlighted by the oval is in keeping with a GIST.

and ulceration. The malignant subtype tends to metastasise to the abdominal cavity and the liver.

Gastric Lymphoma

Stomach involvement in cases of lymphoma can either be secondary (as part of the generalised disease process) or primary, whereby the stomach and regional lymph nodes are predominantly involved. Of the primary subtype, the most common histological variants are diffuse large B cell lymphoma (DLBCL) or lymphoma that has occurred secondary to the presence of mucosal-associated lymphoid tissue (MALT), which itself arises in the most part due to colonisation of the mucosa by *H. pylori*. Gastric lymphoma generally appears as an infiltrative mass on CT and therefore can be mistaken with gastric adenocarcinoma. Some features may be more suggestive of lymphoma, such as diffuse, solid lymphadenopathy. In any case, a biopsy of the gastric lesion is required for definitive characterisation.

THE HEPATOPANCREATOBILIARY SYSTEM

Both CT and MRI are used to characterise diseases of the pancreas and liver. Magnetic resonance cholangiopancreatography (MRCP) is particularly useful to characterise pathologies of the biliary tree.

Acute and chronic pancreatitis are covered in Chapter 2.

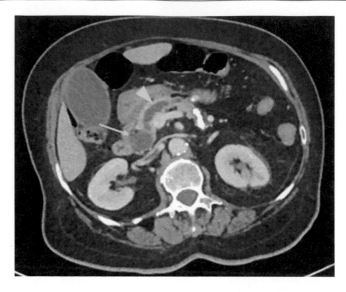

Figure 3.5 Axial CT through the upper abdomen showing dilatation of the CBD (arrow) and pancreatic duct (arrowhead), resulting in the 'double-duct sign'.

Pancreatic and Periampullary Cancer (Ductal Adenocarcinoma)

The aim of imaging in these patients is to identify those with resectable or non-resectable disease to plan surgery only in patients where it is appropriate. US, CT and MRI all have a role in the detection or staging of pancreatic cancer. Tumours of the pancreatic head can obstruct both the pancreatic duct (with associated atrophy of the pancreatic parenchyma) and the common bile duct, resulting in the 'double-duct sign', which can be identified on US (even if the mass itself is difficult to see), as well as on CT (see Figure 3.5) and MRI, whereby the primary tumour may be more reliably seen.

Of the two cross-sectional modalities, dual-phase contrast-enhanced CT in the pancreatic parenchymal as well as the portal venous phases with water ingested as an oral contrast agent is the most common investigation as it is faster and, therefore in many cases, more readily available than MRI. The pancreatic phase preferentially highlights the primary tumour (Figure 3.6a), whereas the delayed portal venous phase better depicts any hepatic, nodal and peritoneal metastases, as shown in Figure 3.6b.

Cystic Tumours of the Pancreas

CT and MRI are used to characterise cystic masses of the pancreas. The most common cystic mass is a pancreatic pseudocyst. True cystic neoplasms include:

- Mucinous cystadenomas, which on imaging comprises a solid mass containing a number of large cystic foci.

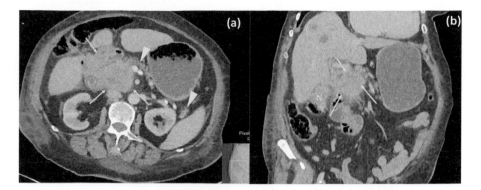

Figure 3.6 (a) Contrast-enhanced axial CT through the upper abdomen showing a large pancreatic head tumour highlighted by arrows. Note the arrowheads depict the normal pancreatic body and tail. (b) Coronal reconstruction showing the pancreatic head tumour (arrows). (N) highlights regional nodal disease and the oval highlights liver metastases.

- Serous cystic tumours comprise multiple small cysts, sometimes with a central scar and/or calcification. MRI may be better at depicting the spongiform, microcystic nature of this lesion.
- Intraductal papillary mucinous neoplasms (IPMNs) arise from the epithelial cells of the ductal system and as such can arise from the main duct or the side branches. Lesions can also be a mixed type arising from both sites. On CT and MRI, IPMNs are characterised by multiple unilocular or septated cystic lesions that communicate with the pancreatic ductal system (Figure 3.7).

Neuroendocrine Tumours (NETs)

In cases of functional NETs, imaging is used to localise the tumour once it is confirmed biochemically. CT is most commonly used and in positive cases shows a hyperenhancing tumour in an early arterial phase scan, with rapid wash-out of the contrast in the portal venous phase, such that the tumour appears of similar density to the surrounding pancreatic parenchyma. The lesions may be solitary (typically in the case of insulinomas) or multiple (typically in the case of gastrinomas). PET-CT using Gallium DOTATATE as a tracer is also helpful to identify NETs.

Non-functioning NETs are almost always malignant and can be difficult to differentiate from pancreatic cancer, save for their avid enhancement (pancreatic cancer usually does not enhance avidly) and the presence of calcification in the mass, which is also not a feature of pancreatic cancer.

Gallbladder Cancer

On imaging these appear as focal or diffuse thickening or intraluminal masses of the gall bladder, which may invade the adjacent structures.

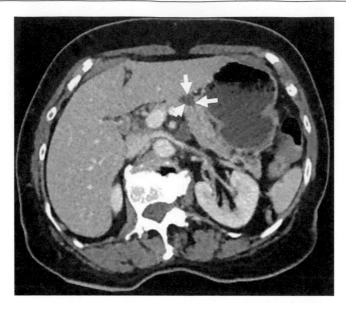

Figure 3.7 Contrast-enhanced axial CT through the upper abdomen. A small cystic lesion of the pancreatic body highlighted by the arrow communicates with the main pancreatic duct and as such is in keeping with an IPMN.

Cholangiocarcinoma

Cholangiocarcinoma can be intrahepatic or more commonly extra-hepatic, and the extrahepatic lesions are subclassified into hilar (proximal to the cystic duct insertion) and distal (distal to the cystic duct insertion) lesions. This classification is based on the TNM staging classification, with a different staging system for each intrahepatic, hilar and distal cholangiocarcinoma.

The macroscopic, and therefore the radiological, appearance of cholangiocarcinomas can be subdivided into three types. In the mass-forming subtype there is a defined hepatic mass. The mass appears of intermediate echogenicity on US and of low attenuation on unenhanced CT. On contrast-enhanced CT and MRI, the mass peripherally enhances in the earlier phases, with 'in-filling'/centripetal enhancement in the later phases.

The periductal infiltrating subtype, where the disease extends along the duct walls, causes proximal bile duct dilatation (see Figure 3.8a). On imaging, the duct wall appears thickened and the duct lumen narrowed, with resultant proximal ductal dilatation.

In cases of the intraductal subtype, the lesion focally proliferates in the duct like a papilliform lesion, which on imaging appears as focal duct ectasia due to the underlying mass, with or without an enhancing underlying intraductal lesion.

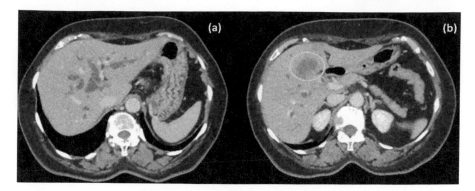

Figure 3.8 Axial CT images of the upper abdomen in the portal venous phase. (a) Intrahepatic ductal dilatation in a case of hilar cholangiocarcinoma. (b) Intrahepatic abscess highlighted with an oval as a complication of the obstructed biliary system.

THE LIVER

US is the workhorse modality to assess the liver and can detect focal lesions, diffuse disease (such as hepatic steatosis and cirrhosis), biliary disease and using Doppler, portal hypertension. Indeterminate hepatic lesions can be further characterised on US using intravenous contrast. US is also used as the main image-guided modality to facilitate histopathological diagnosis by way of transcutaneous core biopsy. The standard abdominal CT contrast phase used to depict most abdominal pathology is the portal venous phase; this phase depicts hepatic lesions such as cysts and metastases well. For indeterminate lesions, other phases (such as early and late arterial and delayed phases) may be required to be performed. MRI has long been used to troubleshoot indeterminate lesions of the liver as various specialised sequences can be implemented to establish their nature. Both generic (gadolinium-based) and hepatobiliary-specific MRI contrast agents can be used.

Liver Metastases

Metastatic lesions of the liver arise from haematogeneous spread. Lesions can appear variable within and across the modalities, but they tend to be multiple and of different sizes at presentation and, in the absence of treatment, tend to grow on serial imaging (see Figure 3.6b).

Primary Liver Cancer

Hepatocellular carcinoma (HCC) is the most common primary malignancy of the liver. Cirrhosis is a common predisposing factor in the development

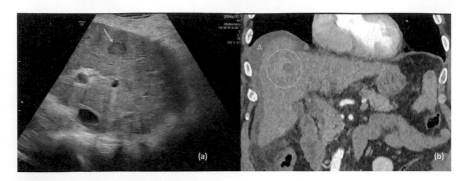

Figure 3.9 (a) US image through the liver showing a solitary focal lesion of the liver (arrow). The background liver echogenicity is abnormal, suggesting micronodules, and the liver edge is irregular, in keeping with cirrhosis. (b) Coronal arterial phase CT through the upper abdomen in the same patient. The hepatic lesion in keeping with HCC in segment VIII of the liver (oval) demonstrates enhancement in the arterial phase, and a small non-enhancing necrotic focus is present at the medial side of the lesion. Note the irregular liver edge in keeping with cirrhosis and the perihepatic ascites (A).

of HCC, and its presence can reduce the sensitivity of imaging to detect smaller lesions in particular. Therefore, a multi-modality approach using US, CT and MRI may be required to establish a likely diagnosis. US contrast and liver-specific MRI contrast agents may also be required to troubleshoot. Lesions can be solitary, multi-focal or diffuse.

HCCs can appear variable on US, hence the need to recommend further imaging in cases of a new lesion that has been detected on US, especially if there are risk factors such as hepatitis B or C or cirrhosis (Figure 3.9a). Indeed, US can be used as a screening tool for HCC in high-risk patients.

Multiphase CT with a late arterial phase is usually required to help characterise HCCs, as most are hypervascular and enhance during the late arterial phase (Figure 3.9b) and demonstrate wash-out in the later portal venous phase. The minority of lesions may contain calcification or fat.

MRI is considered the most sensitive modality for detection of HCC; various sequences as well as the use of liver-specific contrast agents can be implemented.

Fibrolamellar carcinoma (FLC) is considered to be a separate entity to HCC; it tends to occur in younger patients without risk factors. Lesions are usually solitary and well-defined with a central scar that in around half of cases contains calcification, which can help distinguish it from HCC, where calcification is rarer. The unenhanced phase of the CT is useful to look for calcification embedded within the low attenuation scar.

Benign and Cystic Tumours

Hepatic Cysts

Simple hepatic cysts are relatively common and are commonly detected incidentally. They have typical appearances of a thin wall with no soft tissue component and simple fluid content. They can vary in size from tiny to massive and can be multiple.

Hepatic Haemangiomas

These lesions are also commonly encountered incidentally on imaging. On US these appear as well-defined hyperechoic lesions. On contrast-enhanced US, CT and MRI, hepatic haemangiomas typically demonstrate progressive 'centripetal' enhancement, meaning the periphery of the lesion enhances in the earlier arterial phases and the lesion progressively 'fills in' with contrast to its centre in the later portal venous phase.

Focal Nodular Hyperplasia (FNH)

After haemangiomas, this is the most common benign lesion of the liver. A characteristic feature on imaging is the central scar with fibrous septae radiating from it. On contrast-enhanced studies, a large central artery can be seen.

Hepatic Adenomas

These lesions generally remain asymptomatic unless they spontaneously rupture, causing hemorrhage and abdominal pain. They should be considered as hormone-induced tumours, and predisposing factors include oral contraceptive use, anabolic steroids, obesity and diabetes. These lesions are usually solid, large and subcapsular in location. The remainder of the imaging appearances are variable, depending on whether there is intralesional fat or haemorrhage.

REFERENCE

1. Allum WH et al. Gut. (2011). PMID: 21705456.

Chapter 4

Colorectal Surgery

Although endoscopic evaluation is the mainstay of initial assessment of most diseases of the lower gastrointestinal tract, imaging provides essential useful information to guide treatment and to assess treatment response.

COLON CANCER

Colon and rectal cancer can both be managed surgically. Imaging has a vital role in locally staging disease that is amenable to surgical treatment as well as assessing for distant metastases, most commonly to the lymph nodes and the liver.

The two main imaging modalities used in assessment of colon cancer are conventional contrast-enhanced CT and CT colonoscopy (CTC). The latter has replaced barium enemas, which have largely been confined to the radiological archives. On standard CT, malignancy of the colon appears as focal thickening of the bowel wall (Figure 4.1), with or without stranding of the adjacent mesentery, and mesenteric or retroperitoneal nodal enlargement.

Nodularity in the omentum or peritoneum (Figure 4.2) with or without ascites indicates peritoneal disease.

RECTAL CANCER

MRI is used for both local staging of rectal cancer and for assessing response to treatment. On initial assessment, tumour location and characteristics, such as size and regional nodal classification, can be determined. Other MRI-specific characteristics that can be established include depth of invasion, involvement of the sphincter complex and presence of extramural vascular invasion (EMVI).

On T2-weighted MRI images the layers of the rectum can be seen as the mucosa (hypodense), submucosa (hyperdense) and muscularis propria (hypodense). Tumour staging can be assessed with T1 being up to the submucosa, T2 up to the muscularis propria and T3 beyond the muscularis propria

DOI: 10.1201/9781003324362-4

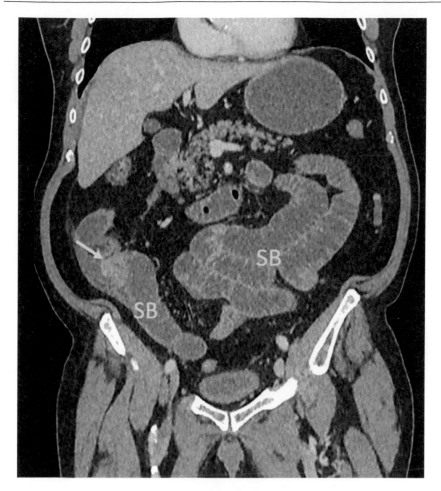

Figure 4.1 Contrast-enhanced coronal CT through the abdomen and pelvis. The arrow highlights an enhancing caecal tumour in the vicinity of the ileocaecal valve. There is secondary obstruction of the small bowel as shown by the dilated small bowel loops, labelled SB.

into the mesorectum. Relying on MRI alone to distinguish between T1 and T2 tumours is not accurate in all cases, and sometimes endoanal ultrasound is required. The anterior peritoneal reflection is seen as the 'seagull sign', which is a hypodense line attached to the anterior wall of the rectum in a V-shape. In tumours that have breeched this margin, T4a tumours, there is a high risk of peritoneal recurrence after surgery.

The anorectal ring should be noted, and the distance between the inferior edge of the tumour and the anorectal ring defines it as a high, mid or low (Figure 4.3) rectal tumour. Low rectal tumours are 0–5 cm from the anal verge, middle 5.1–10 cm and high 10.1–15 cm from the anal verge. Tumours

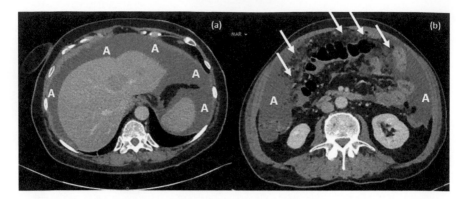

Figure 4.2 Axial contrast-enhanced CT through the upper abdomen. Irregular lesions in the liver in (a) keeping with metastases. Note the malignant ascites (A). (b) The same scan lower in the abdomen showing further ascites as well as omental nodularity (arrows) in keeping with metastatic disease; when it becomes plaque-like as in this case, it is known as 'omental cake'.

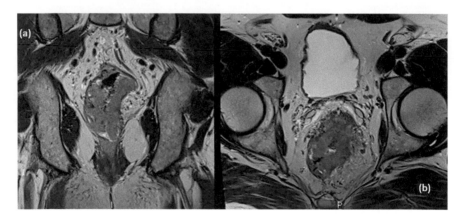

Figure 4.3 Rectal MRI in the same patient. (a) Acquired in the coronal plane and (b) in the axial plane. These images show a bulky, high-risk low rectal cancer with transmural penetration.

located above 15 cm from the anal verge are considered colonic tumours and are managed differently from rectal tumours. On the coronal views the relationship to the internal and external sphincters can be determined to help decide whether sphincter-preserving surgery can be carried out.

Morphology of rectal tumours can also be assessed as polypoidal, circumferential (Figure 4.3), ulcerating or semi-circumferential. They can also be characterised as mucinous or non-mucinous, with mucinous tumours having a higher signal intensity on T2-weighted images, and these also have a poorer prognosis and tend to be more advanced at the time of diagnosis.

The survival of rectal cancer is related to infiltration of the mesorectum and the ability to achieve a negative circumferential resection margin (CRM) at surgery, both factors that MRI can help characterise. The gold standard of treatment for rectal cancer is total mesorectal excision (TME). TME entails complete resection of the mesorectum along the mesorectal fascia (MRF) plane. Neoadjuvant chemoradiation (NCRT) may be given prior to surgical excision with the aim of downstaging disease and minimising local recurrence. MRI identifies tumours that are locally advanced that would benefit from neoadjuvant chemoradiotherapy. The use of NCRT to downstage tumours prior to performing a TME has increased the survival of rectal cancer patients. The MRF is the plane surrounding the mesorectum seen as a low signal intensity line on MRI. In the sagittal plane, the posterior margin of the MRF can be seen in front of the presacral fascia. Within the CRM is the mesorectum, which is the fatty tissue surrounding the rectum containing the lymph nodes and lymphatic vessels. The CRM is defined as the shortest distance between the MRF and tumour, with a distance of less than 1 mm being considered a positive CRM. Between 1–2 mm is considered to be threatening. As noted previously, tumour extending into the mesorectum is classified as T3a and above.

MRI done after NCRT helps assess tumour response, tailor surgical planning and is part of assessment for a complete clinical response (along with digital rectal examination and endoscopic findings). MRI is less accurate at assessing tumours after treatment compared to staging the initial tumour, and a multidisciplinary approach is required using endoscopic and clinical findings. MRI after NCRT may detect colloid degeneration, which is a non-mucinous tumour that becomes mucinous after treatment. This indicates a response to treatment and is a good prognostic sign. In this case it is important to compare pre- and post-treatment images. Fibrosis appears as low intensity signal compared to residual tumour, which is intermediate intensity on T2-weighted images.

MRI is less accurate at assessing lymph node status as opposed to tumour status. The presence of suspicious LNs indicates the need for NCRT, and the presence, location and number should be reported. Regional LNs are mesorectal, superior rectal, middle rectal, inferior rectal, sigmoid mesenteric, inferior mesenteric, lateral sacral, presacral, sacral promontory and internal iliac. LNs outside of these are considered to be distant metastases, M1.

Recurrent Disease

After treatment, MRI is useful for surveillance to detect any recurrence, with the most common site of recurrence being the anastomosis. Imaging is also important for detecting recurrence at other sites that cannot be reached endoscopically or clinically. CT and PET-CT are used for detecting distant recurrence. If recurrence is detected, MRI can help assess resectability and surgical approach in patients undergoing re-excision.

INFLAMMATORY BOWEL DISEASE

Imaging is used to complement endoscopic evaluation in patients with inflammatory bowel disease (IBD). These include the use of CT enterography (CTE), magnetic resonance enterography (MRE) and intestinal ultrasound (IUS). The benefits of imaging are that they provide extra information in the diagnosis, monitoring and detection of complications. Imaging also reduces the need for repeated endoscopic examinations. Although not specific to IBD, bowel wall thickness is a good marker of disease activity, with 3 mm being considered the upper limit of normal. Since chronic inflammation may also lead to bowel wall thickening, other modalities including MRI with gadolinium contrast can be used to look for hyperintense T2 signal in the submucosa as a marker of mucosal oedema seen in severe inflammation. Fat wrapping, which describes the hypertrophy of fat on the mesenteric side, is another useful sign. Ulceration may also be seen in the mucosal layer, both on ultrasound and MRI.

PERIANAL AND RECTAL DISEASE

One of the commonest indications for imaging the perianal region is to investigate perianal sepsis in the acute setting or to investigate for perianal fistulas in patients with recurrent perianal sepsis. Imaging in perianal sepsis is covered in Chapter 2, 'Emergency Surgery'. For perianal fistulae, MRI is usually implemented (Figure 4.4).

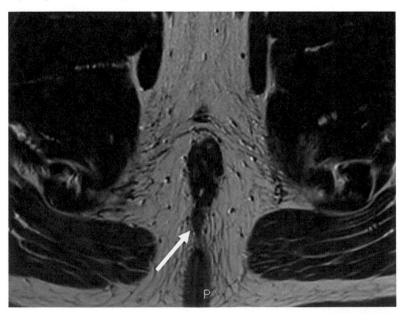

Figure 4.4 Axial T2-weighted image showing a right posterior quadrant intersphincteric fistula at the 6–7 o'clock position (arrow).

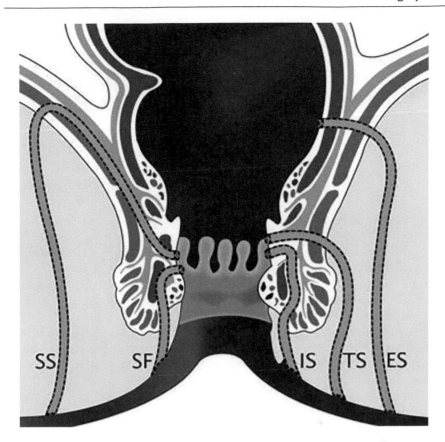

Figure 4.5 Parks Classification. [With permission from (3).]

The original classification by Parks et al. was used to describe the course of the fistula from anal canal to perianal skin in relation to the outermost layer of striated muscle (2).

REFERENCES

1. Rimola J et al. Gut. (2022). PMC 9664122.
2. Parks AG et al. Br J Surg. (1976). PMID: 1267867.
3. Ziech M et al. Clin Gastroenterol Hepatol. (2009). PMID: 19602450.

Chapter 5

Breast Surgery

The primary investigation used to screen or detect breast cancer in symptomatic patients is the mammogram. However, in patients younger than 35 years old, the density of the breast tissue, which appears 'white' on mammogram, can obscure breast lesions; therefore, US is the imaging of choice in these patients. MRI has been established as a problem-solving diagnostic tool because of its high sensitivity in characterising invasive breast cancer.

Percutaneous image-guided biopsy is used to histologically characterise breast lesions. The combination of imaging, clinical examination and needle biopsy, also known as 'triple assessment', is the gold standard for diagnosing breast lesions.

A grading system from the British Society of Breast Radiologists is used to describe the appearances of lesions on mammograms (prefixed with M) and ultrasound (prefixed with U) as follows:

1 Normal
2 Benign
3 Intermediate/probably benign
4 Suspicious for malignancy
5 Highly suspicious of malignancy

The breast is composed mainly of fatty tissue and, unlike other body regions such as the thorax, the breast has a narrow range of inherent densities; therefore, special X-ray equipment is required to produce the low-energy X-rays required for high soft tissue contrast. High spatial resolution is required to identify tiny structures such as microcalcifications, and short exposure times are necessary to ensure sharp images are produced. Abnormal findings on mammograms and US include atypical calcifications and masses. A spiculated mass is usually considered to be highly suspicious.

In this chapter, mammograms will be discussed in more detail, as well as the significance of calcification that may be seen on mammogram. The typical appearances of benign and malignant lesions will also be discussed.

DOI: 10.1201/9781003324362-5

MAMMOGRAMS

Mammograms are performed in two standard views: the mediolateral oblique (MLO) view and the craniocaudal (CC) view (Figure 5.1a,b) with the breast tissue under compression to increase the sensitivity of detection of smaller lesions.

The MLO is the only view in which all the breast tissue is included; a well-positioned MLO projection should include the inframammary angle, the nipple in profile and the nipple level with the caudal end of the pectoralis musculature (see Figure 5.1b).

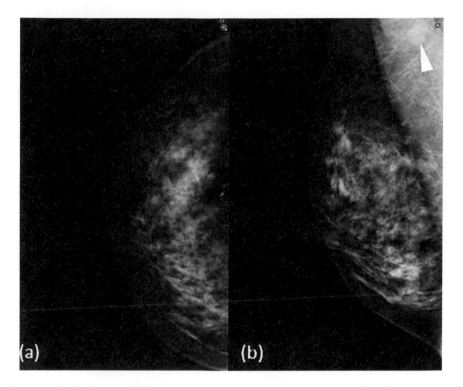

Figure 5.1 (a) Standard CC projection of a normal mammogram. The glandular tissue in the centre of the breast is denser and appears more 'white' on the mammogram. In patients with dense glandular tissue, i.e., younger or lactating patients, this dense glandular tissue can obscure lesions; therefore, US is often used as a first-line modality in symptomatic patients. The 'dark grey' tissue at the periphery is consistent with fatty tissue in the breast. With increasing age, the 'whiter' glandular tissue tends to involute and is replaced by the 'blacker' fatty tissue. This would be reported as M1 (normal). (b) Standard MLO projection of a normal mammogram. The upper chest wall/axilla (top right of the image) is usually visible on this projection, hence a distinction can be made from CC mammograms. As in this case, normal lymph nodes can often be seen in the axilla on the MLO projection (arrowhead). This would be reported as M1 (normal).

A well-positioned CC projection should show the nipple in profile, and it should include all the medial breast tissue and most of the lateral breast tissue apart from the axillary tail (see Figure 5.1a). Further views such as localised targeted compression on 'paddle views' can be obtained; this can result in better separation of tissues to accentuate the appearance of any underlying lesion. Magnification views are usually performed to examine microcalcifications. In patients with silicone and saline implants, the mammographic technique may need to be modified as the implants are usually radiodense and can obscure native breast tissue.

CALCIFICATIONS

Calcification can be identified on US but is usually better characterised on mammography. The distribution of calcification is important to determine whether this is of benign origin or malignant origin (1). The changes in calcification over time are also informative when comparing current with historical mammograms.

Benign Calcification

Rim-like or circumlinear calcifications that line the walls of cysts, known as *tea-cup* calcifications, are in themselves not considered to be malignant.

Popcorn calcification can accumulate within involuting benign lesions such as fibroadenomas, particularly after menopause.

Fat necrosis often presents as *eggshell* calcification or coarse calcification studded within scarring.

Vascular calcifications appear as *tram-lines* that follow the line of vessels within the breast tissue.

Large deposits that follow the course of the ducts and tend to be centered near the nipple are considered benign and occur as a result of disease affecting the mammary ducts. These deposits have a characteristic *broken needle* appearance. If the debris extrudes from the ducts, it can cause an inflammatory reaction that leads to fat necrosis and the so-called lead-pipe appearance on mammography.

Malignant Calcification

Sometimes hazy, poorly defined clusters of microcalcifications occur, which suggests malignancy; therefore, biopsy is usually indicated in these cases. Microcalcification in ductal carcinoma in situ (DCIS) are typically rod-shaped and branched. The greater the number of foci of calcification in an area of DCIS, the greater the risk of invasive disease.

As the presence of calcification may be the only indication of a cancer on mammogram, these need to be interpreted with caution. Magnification of these areas is commonly employed, and if there is any doubt, the lesion should undergo triple assessment, and a percutaneous biopsy as a minimum should be carried out.

BENIGN LESIONS

Simple Cysts

This is the most common cause of a focal breast lesion. Simple cysts have no malignant potential. On mammography, these appear as well-defined dense lesions and ultrasound shows a well-defined, hypoechoic oval or round lesion in the corresponding location with 'posterior acoustic enhancement', equating to brighter-appearing echos beyond the cyst due to the excellent transmission of US waves through the fluid content of the cyst (Figure 5.2). These can be treated at the time of the US with aspiration.

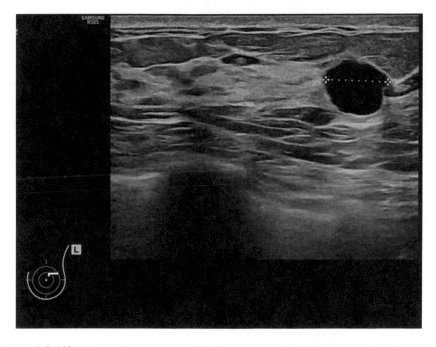

Figure 5.2 US image showing a well-defined completely hypoechoic structure with no internal complexity. Note the brighter signal posterior to the lesion is in keeping with 'posterior acoustic enhancement' due to the excellent transmission of the US waves through the fluid of the cyst.

Fibroadenomas

Fibroadenomas are the most common cause of benign solid lesions in the breast. On mammography, these appear as well-defined rounded or ovoid masses that may contain calcifications, especially in older women.

On US, fibroadenomas are generally hyperechoic with respect to surrounding fat. They are oval-shaped and well-defined, often with a thin echogenic rim. It is important to distinguish fibroadenomas from well-defined carcinomas and phyllodes tumour. This is achieved by percutaneous biopsy as part of the triple assessment.

Papillomas

Papillomas are benign lesions arising in a duct and many can secrete fluid, resulting in nipple discharge clinically. On mammography, these are often seen as a well-defined lesion in a retro areolar location, occasionally with microcalcifications. On US, they appear as a filling defect in a focally dilated duct. The cystic component of the papilloma is often blood-stained on aspiration, aiding in the radiological diagnosis of a papillomatous lesion. Papillomas can contain cellular atypia and therefore a relatively increased risk of malignancy. Furthermore, it is impossible to distinguish papillomas from papillary carcinomas on imaging, so percutaneous biopsy is often required.

Lipomas

These appear as radiolucent masses on mammography and on US usually as well-defined lesions that are septated and hyperechoic with respect to the adjacent subcutaneous fat.

Mastitis and Breast Abscess

US is the usual imaging modality implemented in patients with suspected breast abscess, and findings include an irregular hypoechoic collection that may contain internal echos, associated with oedema (Figure 5.3) and increased reflectivity of the surrounding fat and skin in keeping with cellulitis. Abscesses are usually aspirated by the radiologist under US guidance.

INVASIVE CARCINOMA

Mammography

Carcinomas appear as ill-defined spiculated masses on mammography; the spiculated appearance is usually found in tumours of lower grade and

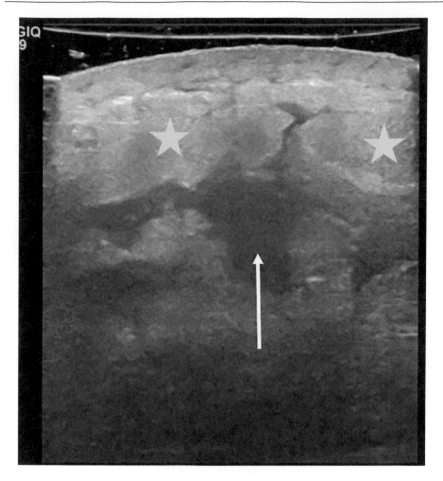

Figure 5.3 US image showing an ill-defined hypoechoic breast collection centrally consistent with abscess (arrow) surrounded by thickening oedema and increased reflectivity of the surrounding fat in keeping with surrounding cellulitis (stars).

is thought to be secondary to the desmoplastic reaction in the surrounding tissue (Figure 5.4). In higher grade poorly differentiated tumours, this desmoplastic reaction may not have had the opportunity to develop, and these lesions may appear better defined and therefore could be mistaken for benign lesions, highlighting the importance of percutaneous biopsy of these lesions.

Ductal carcinoma in situ (DCIS) contains microcalcifications on mammography, and in many cases, invasive ductal carcinoma develops from DCIS, hence the invasive mass can contain these foci of microcalcification. Lobular carcinomas are less likely to be associated with microcalcifications

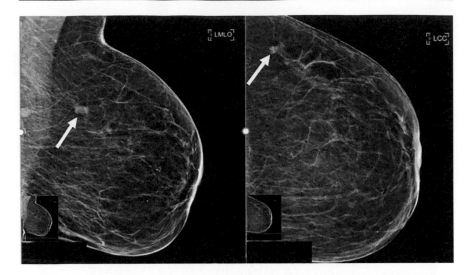

Figure 5.4 Two-view mammography of the left breast showing an ill-defined spiculated lesion at the upper (as shown on the MLO) outer (as shown on
the CC) quadrant highlighted by the arrow is in keeping with invasive
carcinoma of the breast. This lesion is classified as M5.

and are more likely to be apparent as an ill-defined mass or an area of asym-
metrically dense breast tissue. Papillary, medullary and mucinous lesions
may appear as well-defined multi-lobulated lesions that can be mistaken as
benign, hence the importance of carrying out a percutaneous biopsy, even
in cases that are suspected to be benign. Inflammatory breast cancer can
manifest as skin thickening with or without the presence of an underlying
mass.

US

Several characteristic features of malignancy can be demonstrated on US.
Carcinomas are markedly hypoechoic as compared to the surrounding fat;
the lesions typically are larger in their anteroposterior dimension than in
their transverse (left-to-right) dimension, which is sometimes described as
a 'taller-than-wide' appearance; posterior acoustic shadowing is often seen
in the US signal posterior to the lesion, which is due to the inherently high
density of a carcinomatous lesion that tends to block through transmission
of US waves compared to the surrounding tissue (see Figure 5.5).

US is also useful to stage the axilla. Historically, the axilla has been staged
by surgical excision, but pre-operative US can be useful to identify any suspicious lymph nodes that can be targeted pre-operatively with percutaneous
biopsy to determine if the axilla can be surgically spared, saving the patient
from potential co-morbidities such as lymphoedema.

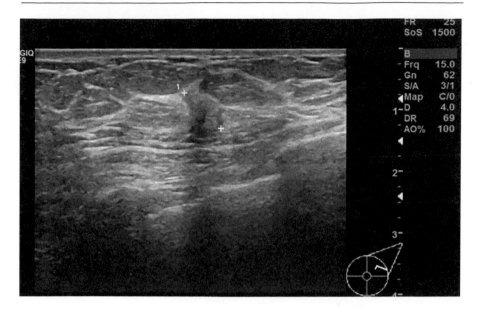

Figure 5.5 US image of the lesion (between the crosses) depicted on the mammogram of Figure 5.6. The lesion is ill-defined, hypoechoic and casts a 'posterior acoustic shadow' due to its dense composition. Note the lesion is 'taller than it is wide', a typical feature of invasive carcinoma on US. It is classified as U5. This lesion is readily amenable to percutaneous biopsy under US guidance.

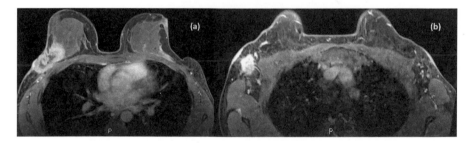

Figure 5.6 (a) Contrast-enhanced breast MRI showing necrotic, fungating right-sided breast cancer. (b) Same MRI showing metastatic nodal disease in the right axilla.

MRI

Contrast-enhanced MRI is becoming increasingly important in the investigation of breast disease, particularly as it has a high sensitivity for detecting invasive breast cancer.

MRI scan is indicated for local staging of breast cancer, screening the younger population where screening may be indicated due to a strong family history of breast cancer and for monitoring the response to neo-adjuvant chemotherapy. Contrast is given to assess enhancement kinetics, such as time to peak enhancement and lesion wash-out (Figure 5.6). Non-contrast MRI can also be helpful to assess the integrity of breast implants.

REFERENCE

1. Nalawade YV. Indian J Radiol Imaging. (2009). PMCID: PMC2797739.

Chapter 6

Vascular Surgery

Imaging modalities used for patients with vascular pathologies include Doppler US, angiography, MR angiogram (MRA), CT angiogram (CTA) and digital subtraction angiography (DSA).

US Doppler mapping of the central and peripheral vessels is operator dependent and, in the UK, tends to be delivered by specialist vascular technicians rather than radiologists. Due to their deep course, assessment of the pelvic veins can be less accurate on US Doppler than with MRA and CTA. The resolution of MRA has improved hugely in recent times, such that it is comparable to CTA, whilst also avoiding the ionising radiation dose; however, some implantable devices such as permanent pacemakers, which are relatively more common in this cohort of patients, can pose a challenge to imaging on some MRI scanners. MRA usually takes significantly longer than CTA to perform, so CTA can be more efficient in patients with pain who struggle to keep still for long periods to perform the imaging on a CT scanner rather than on an MRI scanner. Interventional radiology (IR) has certainly taken on a much more significant role in the management of vascular conditions. Using minimally invasive techniques and image guidance, commonly in the form of DSA, interventional radiologists are able to treat many vascular conditions, including those that present acutely such as critical limb ischaemia, as well as more chronic conditions such as intermittent claudication. DSA better visualises enhanced vessels than conventional fluoroscopy as the initial pre-contrast fluoroscopic image (known as the mask) is 'subtracted' from the post-contrast fluoroscopic image, creating a crisper image of the enhanced vessels.

In this chapter the common imaging techniques used are described in more detail. For ease, imaging modalities have been divided into arterial and venous studies.

PERIPHERAL ARTERIAL DISEASE

Clinical presentation of arterial disease ranges from intermittent claudication to critical limb ischaemia complicated by gangrene or ulceration

DOI: 10.1201/9781003324362-6

indicating tissue loss. Management of patients and urgency of intervention is determined by the performance status, clinical presentation and the radiological findings.

Ultrasound, Including Duplex and Doppler Scans

Blood flow can be qualitatively assessed using colour on the US machine and quantitatively assessed using spectral Doppler waveforms by assessing the frequency of the sound waves returned to an US transducer; these represent the heterogeneous Doppler shifts produced by each red blood cell in motion, each of which has a unique velocity. A mathematical model known as Fourier analysis averages the frequencies over a defined time period. These frequencies are converted into velocities using another mathematical model, the Doppler equation. These velocities are then displayed as colour in the vessels/tissue, and a Doppler waveform on the image can also be generated.

An arterial duplex scan (so called because it combines the greyscale image of the US with the Doppler information) involves Doppler ultrasound assessment of the arteries to assess the location and degree of any vascular stenosis. This is facilitated by measuring the peak systolic velocity (PSV) and end diastolic velocity (EDV) of the blood flowing along the length of an artery. The PSV and EDV vary depending on the function of the type of vessel being examined. Low-resistance vessels such as the internal carotid and renal arteries supply organs that require blood flow throughout the cardiac cycle, and these vessels therefore exhibit a high EDV. High-resistance vessels such as the limb arteries are physiologically characterised by low or non-existent EDV.

The localised reduction of the diameter in stenotic arteries increases resistance to blood flow, causing increased PSV and EDV distal to the stenosed site; the high velocity results in turbulent flow, in turn causing spectral broadening on the Doppler examination. To an extent, the greater the stenosis, the greater the PSV and EDV. In very marked stenoses that result in near occlusion, flow velocity is usually unreliable due to the altered haemodynamics. In complete occlusion, PSV and EDV are absent. An example of an arterial US Doppler in a healthy versus an abnormal lower limb is shown in Figure 6.1.

Once the arterial vessels in question have been examined, a report is generated mapping the findings anatomically (Figure 6.2).

CT Angiogram (CTA)

CT angiogram allows assessment of the vasculature using iodinated contrast (Figure 6.3). Timing of scan acquisition in relation to administration of contrast is critical in obtaining accurate images. CT angiogram is essential

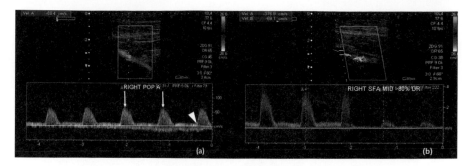

Figure 6.1 (a) Arterial duplex examination in a healthy lower limb. Note the Doppler scale unit is cm/s. The arrows depict the PSV, which is in the normal range for this vessel (around 60 cm/s) and stable throughout the study. The arrowhead depicts the EDV, which arises before the upshoot of systole in the next cardiac cycle; note the low EDV as is expected in this relatively high-resistance vessel. The single colour of red in the vessel highlights the average flow in this vessel is homogeneous and in one direction. (b) Duplex US showing a stenoesed superficial femoral artery. Note the Doppler scale unit is m/s. The PSV is significantly higher at almost 4 m/s (orders of magnitude higher than in the previous physiological example). The EDV is also significantly increased. The varied colours representing flow in the vessel relate to the turbulence of the flow.

in the pre-procedural planning of radiological interventions and surgical procedures as it helps not only to choose the most suitable procedure, but also to plan vascular access.

Magnetic Resonance Angiography (MRA)

MR angiography (Figure 6.4) is useful as it can provide a more detailed assessment of plaque morphology, but it is not always available, and some patients may not be suitable candidates for MRI due to claustrophobia or having implantable devices in situ.

Conventional and Digital Subtraction Angiography (DSA)

Unlike US, CTA and MRA, this is an invasive examination that requires cannulation of the arteries to acquire the image. As well as for diagnostic purposes, angiography is performed in the context of intervention being required, for example, balloon angioplasty of a stenosed superficial femoral artery, as shown in Figure 6.5.

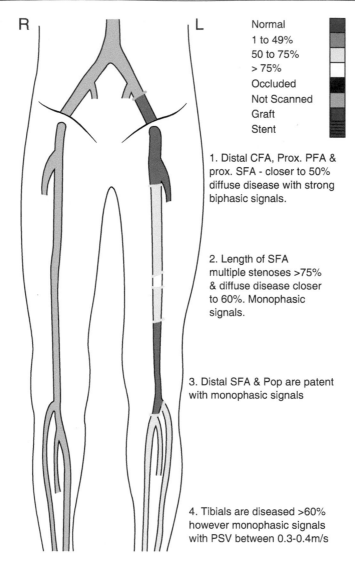

Normal
1 to 49%
50 to 75%
> 75%
Occluded
Not Scanned
Graft
Stent

1. Distal CFA, Prox. PFA & prox. SFA - closer to 50% diffuse disease with strong biphasic signals.

2. Length of SFA multiple stenoses >75% & diffuse disease closer to 60%. Monophasic signals.

3. Distal SFA & Pop are patent with monophasic signals

4. Tibials are diseased >60% however monophasic signals with PSV between 0.3-0.4m/s

Figure 6.2 An example of an arterial duplex scan report, whereby a pictorial representation of the location and extent of stenoses are depicted in an infographic for ease of reference for the vascular surgeon.

EMBOLIC AND THROMBOTIC ARTERIAL OCCLUSIVE DISEASE

In patients presenting with acute ischaemia, the viability of the limb will determine the most appropriate investigation, with immediately threatened limbs undergoing investigation with catheter angiography and possible intervention.

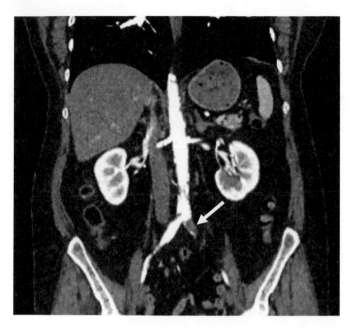

Figure 6.3 Arterial phase coronal CT. The aorta and the right common iliac vessels are opacified by contrast. Note the 'nodular' appearance at the arterial walls is in keeping with deposits of atheromatous plaques. The proximal left common iliac artery does not enhance as well as the right side due to dense atheromatous plaque deposition (arrow).

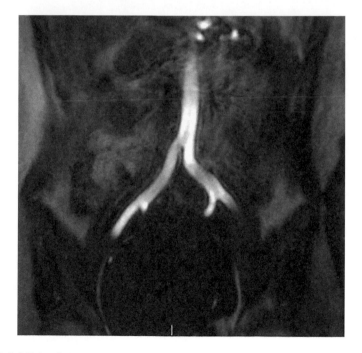

Figure 6.4 MRA of the aorta and iliac vessels.

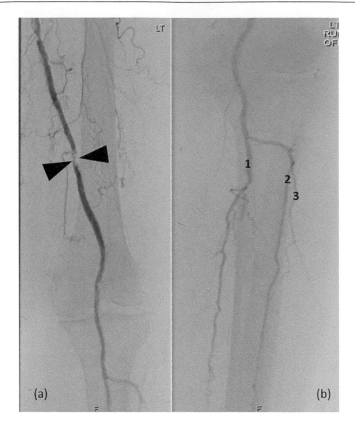

Figure 6.5 DSA of the left lower limb. (a) Shows focal occlusion in the SFA from an atherosclerotic plaque, highlighted by the arrowheads. Note the collateral vessels proximal to the occlusion. (b) Demonstrates intact three-vessel run-off (1 = posterior tibial artery, 2 = anterior tibial artery, 3 = peroneal artery).

For patients with marginally threatened limbs, CTA is more appropriate, but for practical reasons, CTA is also usually performed in cases of critical limb ischaemia. Imaging can help to determine not only the location of any lesions but also the morphology. Arterial thrombosis is usually seen as a sharp or tapered cutoff on arteriography. Diffuse atherosclerosis with well-developed collateral circulation is generally present (well depicted in Figure 6.5a). An embolus will often demonstrate a sharp cutoff with a rounded reverse meniscus sign. The embolus may also be visible as an intraluminal filling defect if the vessel is not completely occluded. Other findings that are most consistent with an embolus include the presence of otherwise normal vessels, the absence of collateral circulation and the presence of multiple filling defects.

If thrombolysis is being considered, performing catheter angiography directly reduces the contrast load for the patient. In patients who have had previous intervention such as stenting or who are known to have atherosclerosis, it is always useful to compare any previous imaging to new imaging.

ABDOMINAL AORTIC ANEURYSM (AAA)

AAAs are commonly identified incidentally on CT as well as in symptomatic cases. The caliber of the abdominal aorta should be routinely checked during an abdominal US examination by the radiologist or sonographer in all patients over the age of 40. The anteroposterior diameter of the aneurysm is recorded as the diameter for surgical planning purposes, usually with a 5.5 cm cutoff in men for consideration of referral for intervention to the vascular surgeon. CTA (Figure 6.6) provides a much more detailed assessment of the morphology of an aortic aneurysm, the surrounding anatomy and helps to plan treatment, including the suitability of endovascular aneurysm repair (EVAR) as well as planning the type of grafts that should be used, for example, whether a fenestrated graft is required. It is also useful to look for the presence of atherosclerotic disease elsewhere, which is also important in deciding which type of graft may be required. CTA including an unenhanced abdominal CT should be performed in cases of suspected aneurysm rupture (see following section). CTA is also used in patients not meeting the criteria for treatment but who require surveillance. It is also used for monitoring complications in patients who have had treatment.

Emergency Aneurysmal Disease

Ultrasound scan is used in the elective setting to diagnose or screen for aneurysmal disease. While ultrasound scan confirms the presence of an ectatic aorta or aneurysm, it will not identify a leak. This is best done with CT abdomen with arterial contrast, which shows haemorrhage in the retroperitoneum (Figure 6.7). The presence of an aortic filling defect represents intraluminal thrombus.

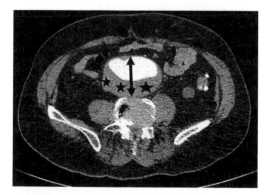

Figure 6.6 Contrast-enhanced axial CT in the arterial phase. A large AAA contains a crescent of thrombus (stars), predominantly sited posteriorly. Note the bright contrast filling the remainder of the lumen. The double-headed arrow highlights the anteroposterior diameter of the AAA, which is the measurement the radiologist provides to the surgeon as the true diameter.

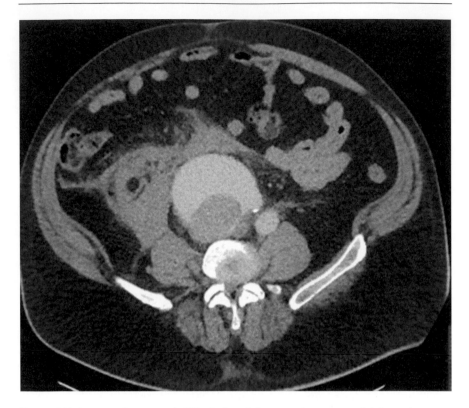

Figure 6.7 Aortic phase axial CT of the abdomen showing an AAA, with retro-peritoneal haemorrhage is in keeping with rupture. Note the intraluminal filling defect in keeping with thrombus.

TRANSIENT ISCHAEMIC ATTACKS (TIAs) AND CEREBROVASCULAR ACCIDENT (CVA)/STROKE

Doppler US is the first-line investigation of TIAs. As with peripheral vascular lesions elsewhere, the Doppler is used to quantify the peak systolic velocity (PSV) values but also looks at plaque morphology. The intima media thickness (IMT) can also be measured on Doppler and is thought to be a predictor of coronary and cerebrovascular events (1); it is seen as two relatively echogenic lines in the vessel wall separated by a hypoechoic area. It is also important to identify near occlusion, as these patients are less likely to benefit from carotid endarterectomy.

Patients presenting acutely with CVA/stroke should ideally be directed towards a specialist stroke centre (2), where they will be referred immediately for unenhanced CT brain and head and neck CTA. The unenhanced CT brain has a secondary purpose of confirming hyperacute stroke, which should be diagnosed clinically by the stroke physician, as the radiological signs can be very subtle early on. Rather, the main purpose of this CT is to assess for any intracranial haemorrhage (see Chapter 10), which is a contraindication to thrombolysis. The purpose of the CTA is to establish if there is a filling defect amenable to thrombectomy, which is performed by radiologists in the neuro-interventional suite.

VENOUS DISEASE

Duplex ultrasonography has become the gold standard investigation for assessing the veins. It allows for both anatomical and haemodynamic assessment of the venous system to identify reflux and thromboses (Figure 6.8). The vascular technician service performs the mapping and dynamic assessment for varicosities using duplex scans in the UK. Various maneuvers are implemented to extenuate the abnormal veins, including scanning the patient in the standing position, compression of the vein with the probe (normally the vein obliterates with mild compression, if the lumen contains thrombus the vein does not obliterate), and compression of the calf; the latter normally produces reflux into more proximal vessels, which is picked up on the Doppler examination. Greater than 0.5 m/s of reverse flow is considered to be pathological reflux, and in the deep veins, absence of reflux is in keeping with DVT. In the case of a patient who presents with a swollen leg, US can also readily pinpoint differential diagnoses such as cellulitis (suggested by reactive inguinal lymph nodes and subcutaneous oedema) and a ruptured Baker's cyst.

Conventional venography under fluoroscopy is no longer performed. CTV and MRV don't have a role in assessing varicose veins but can be

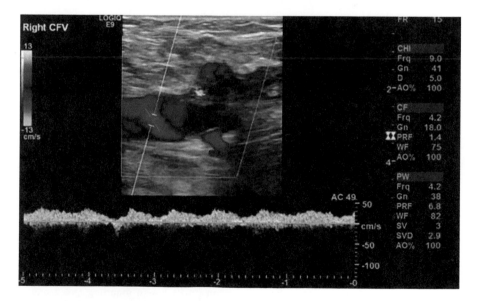

Figure 6.8 Duplex US of the right lower limb. Focal absence of Doppler signal in the right common femoral vein. Note the normal Doppler signal in the remainder of the vessel where there is no thrombus.

useful for the central veins and deep veins, respectively, which can be technically difficult to assess with ultrasound.

DISEASES OF THE LYMPHATICS

Pathological lymph nodes in the neck, axilla and groins are very well visualised with US and they tend to appear enlarged and rounded, rather than ovoid in morphology. The central echogenic sinus, which is well seen in normal lymph nodes, can be obliterated in pathological nodes. Pathological nodes can also be hypervascular, especially in the case of lymphoma. A final feature of pathological nodes is necrosis. This can be caused by infection, for example, tuberculosis. Squamous cell carcinoma that has metastasised to lymph nodes also causes necrosis. Pathological nodes detected on US can be targeted for US-guided biopsy for definitive histopathological diagnosis. PET-CT/PET-MRI can also be used to identify metabolically active lymph nodes (Figure 6.9), which depending on their 'intensity', quantified as the standardised uptake values (SUVs), which can either be reactive/inflammatory or pathological.

A nuclear medicine study known as lymphoscintigraphy (Figure 6.10a,b) is commonly used to image the lymphatic system (3). A labelled isotope in the form of[99] Technitium is injected into the peripheral tissue, and due to the lymphatic drainage and after some time, the lymphatic network can be detected by imaging using a gamma camera to produce a 2D image of the lymphatic network. Three-dimensional imaging is also possible using Single Photon Emission Computed Tomography (SPECT). SPECT-CT combines the 3D map with conventional CT to improve the anatomical resolution of mapping the lymphatic tree.

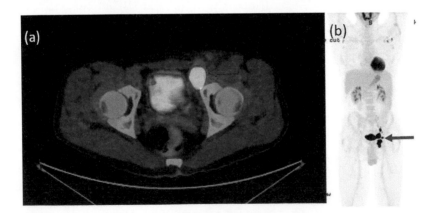

Figure 6.9 (a) Axial PET/CT at the level of the pelvis showing FDG avid nodal disease secondary to non-Hodgkin's lymphoma in the left inguinal region. (b) Maximum intensity projection (MIP) image mapping the areas of increased FDG uptake in a single screenshot. The red arrow labels the pathological left pelvic and inguinal lymph nodes. Note the physiological uptake in the urinary bladder, kidneys, liver and heart.

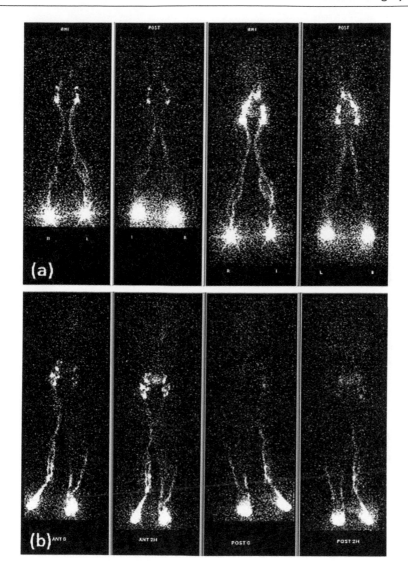

Figure 6.10 (a) Lymphoscintigram in a patient with normal lymphatic drainage. (b) Lymphoscintigram in another patient shows reduced activity in the left thigh in keeping with sluggish lymphatic drainage.

REFERENCES

1. Saba L et al. Atherosclerosis. (2012). PMID: 21968317.
2. Sentinel Stroke National Audit Programme. (2023). www.strokeaudit.org/SupportFiles/Documents/Guidelines/NOSIP-master-version.aspx.
3. Munn LL, Padera TP. Microvasc Res. (2014). PMCID: PMC4268344.

Chapter 7

Paediatric Surgery

All of the imaging modalities have a place in diagnosing pathology in the paediatric cohort, but extra caution is required when considering the use of CT in particular as children are more sensitive than adults to radiation due to the increased radiosensitivity of their developing organs and because they have a relatively longer life span to accumulate exposure and for any deleterious effects of the radiation to manifest.

US is heavily utilised in children to avoid issues related to radiation exposure and because their relatively smaller bodies means a superior view of deep structures, for example, those in the abdomen and pelvis, can often be imaged satisfactorily without the use of CT or MRI. Fluoroscopy is another modality commonly utilised by paediatric radiologists, including in the emergency situations of suspected intussusception and malrotation.

The paediatric population can present diagnostic challenges to the surgeon as this is a heterogeneous population where disease can be age-dependent. Younger children tend to be poor historians, and common symptoms, such as vomiting and abdominal pain, tend to be vague; therefore, imaging may be required to unlock the diagnosis. Common causes of abdominal pain in children are as follows (1):

Infants and toddlers

Gastroenteritis
Intussusception
Mesenteric adenitis
Renal pathology
Malrotation
Abdominal malignancy
Meckel's diverticulum

Toddlers to adolescents

Appendicitis
Mesenteric adenitis
Inflammatory bowel disease

DOI: 10.1201/9781003324362-7

Bowel obstruction
Renal pathology
Ovarian pathology
Abdominal malignancy
Pancreatitis
Distal ileal obstruction syndrome
Meckel's diverticulum

The first-line imaging modality in the majority of cases of abdominal pain is either plain film or US. Non-bilious and bilious vomiting need to be distinguished. The presence of green bilious vomiting must always be investigated urgently to exclude a malrotation. If not detected early, this can lead to significant bowel infarction and death.

CHILDHOOD ABDOMINAL EMERGENCIES

Acute Appendicitis

Acute appendicitis is the most common condition requiring surgery in children but is an uncommon condition in children under three years old, likely due to the funnel shape of the appendix in this cohort. Young children with appendicitis can present late due to an unclear history and, as a result, perforation and appendicular abscess formation are more common in this age group. The late presentation of appendicitis with abscess formation may even lead to small bowel obstruction.

Ultrasound scan is usually the imaging of choice and may show a distended appendix over 6 mm in diameter. There may be associated small bowel ileus, free fluid or abscess. In late cases, portal pyaemia may be detected as air in the portal venous system, which can be well seen on US. When diagnostic uncertainty still persists after US, CT scan may be indicated. The appearances of appendicitis on US and CT has been described in Chapter 2.

Mesenteric Adenitis

One of the differentials of acute appendicitis, this condition may also cause acute abdominal pain and raised inflammatory markers. Ultrasound is useful as it can detect abnormally large mesenteric lymph nodes greater than 10 mm in diameter. There may be increased numbers of nodes, with no other abnormal findings.

Intussusception

Intussusception occurs when a proximal segment of bowel, the intussusceptum, prolapses and invaginates into another distal (receiving) segment, the intussuscipiens. It typically occurs in patients between three and nine months who usually present with colicky abdominal pain indicated by drawing up of the legs into the abdomen, as well as red currant jelly stool.

Intussusception commonly occurs secondary to inflammation of Peyer's patches during a viral infection, such as an upper respiratory tract infection. Other lead points are rare and include Meckel's diverticulum and bowel lymphoma. The most common pattern of intussusception is ileo-colic, which occurs in 90% of cases. Ileo-ileal, colo-colic, ileo-ileo-colic may also occur.

Along with malrotation, intussusception is one of the two paediatric emergencies that warrant emergency radiological investigation and intervention. The patient should be managed in a paediatric surgical centre to ensure rapid assessment, stabilisation and surgical invention if radiological intervention fails.

Ultrasound scan is the initial investigation and has almost 100% diagnostic accuracy. In positive cases, this shows a 'target' or 'doughnut' sign in the transverse plane due to a hypoechoic outer ring formed by oedematous small bowel surrounding a hyperechoic centre, which represents mucosa and intraluminal content (Figure 7.1a). In the longitudinal section this gives a 'pseudokidney' appearance (Figure 7.1c). Poor Doppler flow to the segment predicts a higher failure rate with non-surgical treatment.

Once intussusception is confirmed on US, the patient is immediately transferred to the fluoroscopy suite for an air enema, which is performed by the radiologist with the support of the paediatric surgeon. A control fluoroscopic image is taken to assess for pneumoperitoneum, which is an absolute contraindication to continuing with the procedure. A rectal tube is passed and secured, and air is insufflated into the bowel at a controlled pressure (usually ranging between 80–120 mmHg), with simultaneous fluoroscopic monitoring of the bowel gas pattern to assess for a sudden change in the bowel gas pattern with air entering the small bowel, indicating success.

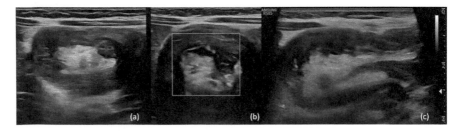

Figure 7.1 US in a child with an ileo-colic intussusception. (a) The typical 'doughnut sign'. (b) Blood flow in the bowel of the intussusception. Poor Doppler flow to the segment predicts a higher failure rate with non-surgical treatment. (c) The transverse US view of the intussusception demonstrating the 'pseudokidney' appearance. (Images courtesy of Dr Trevor Gaunt.)

Continuous fluoroscopic monitoring is essential to establish if a perforation has occurred during the procedure, in which case the rectal insufflation is abandoned and the patient is taken to the operating theatre.

Hemolytic Uraemic Syndrome (HUS)

This is mentioned here as it is a cause of acute abdominal pain in children and has a similar presentation to intussusception. It occurs after gastroenteritis caused by *E. coli* 0157:117, causing acute renal failure. Patients present with abdominal pain, vomiting, fever and bloody stool, and US is used to differentiate this condition from intussusception. In the case of HUS, US shows thickening of the bowel wall and free fluid without the 'doughnut' and 'pseudokidney' signs seen in intussusception.

Malrotation

Malrotation may present acutely with abdominal pain and bilious vomiting. This condition occurs when the bowel does not rotate and fix normally as it returns into the abdominal cavity during embryological development. This abnormality predisposes the child to midgut volvulus around the superior mesenteric artery, which may cause compromise to the blood supply of the small and large bowel, leading to high morbidity and mortality.

All patients in which this is suspected should be referred to a paediatric surgical centre and, once there, be referred to a radiologist to undergo a gastrograffin meal (Figure 7.2) in order to locate the position of the DJ flexure. This is the second paediatric emergency in which emergency radiological input is required (the other being intussusception).

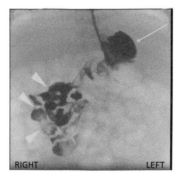

Figure 7.2 Fluoroscopic study where water-soluble contrast has been instilled via the NG tube. The arrow shows contrast in the stomach. The duodenum, DJ flexure and jejunum have been opacified and are all sited to the right of the midline (arrowheads), in keeping with malrotation. (Image courtesy of Dr Trevor Gaunt.)

Under fluoroscopic guidance, water-soluble contrast is instilled into the NG tube, and is traced into the proximal small bowel. Normally, the DJ flexure lies to the left of the midline at the level of L3 or above. In malrotation, the DJ flexure lies on the right (Figure 7.2). Fluoroscopic confirmation of the diagnosis necessitates prompt surgical intervention.

Overall, radiology plays a unique role in the diagnosis and treatment of paediatric surgical conditions. Hence the role of the paediatric radiologist is undertaken by a specially trained radiologist dedicated to paediatrics, who is supported by the paediatric surgeon, should surgery be required.

REFERENCE

1. Carty H. Eur Radiol. (2002). 12:2835–2848. PMID: 12439562.

Chapter 8

Urology

US, CT and MRI all have uses in the diagnosis of urological conditions. Assessment of the genitourinary tract forms a standard part of an abdominal ultrasound scan and may lead to the incidental findings of congenital anomalies.

COMMON CONGENITAL ANOMALIES

These anomalies can be considered according to their anatomical locations.

Kidney

These conditions are usually well depicted on US as well as cross-sectional imaging (CT/MRI) and include the following.

Renal Agenesis

This is associated with absence of the ipsilateral ureter or the presence of a ureteric stump. An absence of the ipsilateral adrenal gland occurs in 10% of cases. Bilateral agenesis results in Potter syndrome and oligohydramnios, pulmonary hypoplasia and distinct facies.

Supernumerary Kidney

This is rare, and when it does occur it is more common on the left side and inferior to the native kidney, either drained by a bifid single left ureter or a complete duplication and a separate second ureter.

Ectopic Kidney

Commonly occurs more inferiorly than the native kidney and can be located in the iliac fossae or pelvis. Pelvic kidneys are more prone to stone formation and vesico-ureteric reflux.

DOI: 10.1201/9781003324362-8

Horseshoe Kidney

These have a two-to-one male-to-female preponderance and are more prone to stone formation and ureteropelvic junction obstruction. There is an increased incidence of anal, cardiovascular and genital abnormalities and increased risk of tumours including Wilms.

Crossed Fused Ectopia

One kidney (more commonly the left) crosses the midline to fuse with the contralateral side. This is a distinct entity from horseshoe kidney, as in this condition both kidneys are at one side of the midline.

Ureter

Fluoroscopy is often used to assess the number and course of the ureters, as well as to establish if there is any structural abnormality such as ureteric stricture, dilatation and hydronephrosis.

Abnormal Ureteric Number

This can consist of bifid collecting systems comprising two renal pelvises or two entirely separate ureters. Two renal pelvises become symptomatic when urine refluxes from one ureter into the other, suspected when one ureteric component is enlarged and if the renal parenchyma being drained appears atrophic/scarred. When there is complete duplication of the ureter, the ureter draining the upper moiety tends to insert ectopically into the bladder (medial and inferior to the normal VUJ). It follows therefore that if the upper urinary tract is abnormal, its draining ureter is likely to have a dysplastic insertion. The ectopic ureter often strictures, resulting in ureterocele formation. The ureter draining the lower moiety inserts normally but can reflux, causing lower pole hydronephrosis. The consistency of the upper and lower moieties draining via their respective duplicitous (ectopic and native) ureters is known as the Weigert-Meyer rule.

Abnormal Ureteric Location

This is usually due to extra-ureteric anatomical causes such as retroperitoneal fibrosis, retroperitoneal lymphadenopathy or vascular aneurysms.

Abnormal Ureteric Calibre

Ureteric strictures can be congenital and are thought to be acquired due to ischaemia in utero. Ureteric dilatation could be due to abnormal ureteric musculature that inhibits peristalsis and causes upstream dilatation.

Vesicoureteric Reflux (VUR)

This condition increases the risks of renal infection and eventual scarring, and is the most common cause of antenatal hydronephrosis. The severity or grade of VUR is determined using the fluoroscopic study of voiding cysto-urethrography (VCUG).

Bladder

Congenital bladder abnormalities can be well seen on US and cross-sectional imaging studies.

Agenesis

In this very rare condition, the ureters normally insert ectopically.

Bladder Diverticula

These are often incidental and asymptomatic but can predispose to stone formation and infection. When present at the VUJ (commonly causing VUR), this is known as a Hutch diverticulum. A bladder ear is an entity whereby the bladder diverticulum descends into the internal inguinal ring.

Prune-belly syndrome is another rare condition consisting of absent rectus abdominis muscles, thin and lax anterior abdominal wall, undescended testes, dilated ureter and prostatic urethra and abnormal kidneys. The bladder wall is usually thickened and the urachus is usually patent.

Urethra

Fluoroscopic studies are the mainstay of assessment of congenital urethral pathologies.

Posterior Urethral Valves

The most common malformation of the urethra occurs when there is a raised mucosal fold that arises between the verumontanum (the boundary between the membranous and prostatic urethra) and the caudal prostatic urethra. This is often diagnosed in the context of bilateral hydronephrosis. On VCUG, the valve may not be seen, but the secondary features of a dilated and lengthened posterior urethra can be seen.

RENAL MASSES

Patients can be referred for imaging if they present with symptoms or signs suggesting a renal mass such as a haematuria or a palpable mass per se.

A relatively common indication for further imaging is a mass that is detected on imaging performed for some other reason, for example, on an abdominal US in which a solid renal lesion is incidentally identified.

Renal masses are best characterised by cross-sectional imaging based on their enhancement characteristics; namely, a malignant lesion such as renal cell carcinoma (RCC) will typically exhibit enhancement. It follows therefore that a non-contrast (control) study is performed initially (Figure 8.1a), contrast is then given, and a second contrast-enhanced CT is performed in the nephrographic phase (Figure 8.1b). In some centres, an intermediate phase known as the corticomedullary phase is also performed and can be useful to assess for the presence of pseudotumours and also to assess the renal vein. The difference in density of the lesion (measured as Hounsfield units, HUs) between the unenhanced and contrast-enhanced studies is determined, and if there is a difference of greater than 20 HUs between the control and the nephrographic phases, the lesion is highly likely to be neoplastic. Care must be taken to measure the density of the solid portion of the lesion, excluding any cystic component, and the same portion of the lesion should be examined between the CT phases. Benign lesions such as simple cysts will not enhance. Renal oncocytomas and renal cell carcinomas can have similar enhancement characteristics on CT; therefore, differentiating them using this modality alone can be tricky. A helpful differentiating feature of oncocytomas on CT that is sometimes present is a central scar, which is less common in RCC. In any case, there will be a low threshold for biopsy in

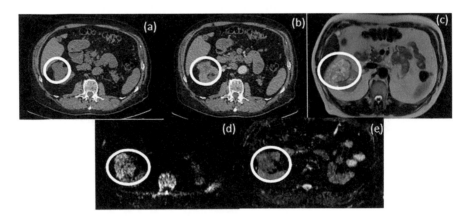

Figure 8.1 Renal mass protocol CT. Oval outlines the lesion described. (a) Axial unenhanced image showing an irregular exophytic lesion arising from the upper pole of the right kidney. (b) Axial contrast-enhanced study that shows the lesion clearly enhances, there is more than a 20 HU difference in the density between the lesions as depicted in (a) and (b). (c) Axial T2-weighted MRI of the lesion, and (d) and (e) are the DWI and ADC maps, showing the lesion restricts diffusion in keeping with a malignancy.

these patients. Assessment of the renal vein for tumour thrombus is important for staging purposes.

MRI with contrast can also be used to assess lesion enhancement. Different MRI sequences can be performed to emphasise certain tissues such as fat or fluid (in the case of cystic foci and angiomyolipomas), and when used in combination with contrast enhancement, lesion nature can be determined. Diffusion-weighted imaging (DWI) and its counterpart sequence, the apparent diffusion coefficient (ADC) map, are helpful to distinguish benign from malignant entities (Figure 8.1d,e). DWI is a method of signal contrast generation based on the differences in Brownian motion. ADC is a measure of the magnitude of diffusion (of water molecules) within tissue. Malignant lesions tend to 'restrict diffusion' and show high intensity on DWI and corresponding low intensity on the ADC map. MRI has an important place in the surveillance imaging of those patients with conditions predisposing them to renal malignancy, such as Von Hippel-Lindau disease, as these patients would otherwise be exposed to a high cumulative radiation dose over their lifetimes with CT.

It is also helpful to assess the coronal plane on CT and MRI as this plane gives a good indication of the extent of a lesion.

Cystic Lesions

Cystic lesions should be characterised on imaging according to the Bosniak classification (Table 8.1), with increasing levels of complexity such as wall

Table 8.1 Table of Bosniak Classification of Renal Cysts (1)

Category	Description	Malignancy Risk
I	Simple cyst; fluid density, hairline wall, no septa calcification or solid components, no enhancement post-IV contrast	0%
II	Cyst with some hairline septa, fine calcification or short segment of thickened calcification Uniformly high-density lesions (<3 cm) No enhancement	<5%
IIF	Multiple hairline thin septa Minimal smooth thickening of wall or septa 'Perceived' enhancement of septa or wall No measurable enhancement Thick nodular calcification in wall/septa Uniformly high-density lesions (>3 cm)	Approx. 20%
III	Thickened, irregular smooth enhancing walls or septa	Approx. 50%
IV	Characteristics of category III lesions with additional soft tissue components independent of the walls/septa	Approx. 90%

nodularity or calcifications being more often associated with malignancy. This classification is strictly speaking a CT-based system, but US is often adequate to classify Bosniak I cysts. Bosniak IIF and above cysts require further assessment, either with imaging follow-up or biopsy, depending on the category. No further management is required for Bosniak category I and II cysts.

CT Urogram

Urothelial malignancies such as transitional cell carcinoma (TCC) are usually suspected in cases of haematuria, and these are best characterised on a CT urogram (CTU), usually once nephrogenic causes, such as glomerulonephritis, have been excluded. CTU entails imaging the kidneys and collecting systems in three phases. A pre-contrast phase is carried out to look for renal stones and as a baseline to assess contrast enhancement of any lesions. A nephrographic phase is performed to characterise any renal lesions that are present (and possibly causing the symptoms). Finally, a delayed pyelographic (excretory) phase, whereby the contrast is imaged once it has been excreted into the collecting system, is performed; this final phase can be considered to be akin to the now largely redundant intravenous urograms (IVUs) (Figure 8.2). The location of filling defects identified on the urographic phase should be compared to the same location on the nephrographic phase, where if the lesion is big enough it may be able to be discretely identified against the low attenuation of the urine (fluid density of around 0 HU) in the collecting systems.

URINARY CALCULUS DISEASE

Imaging patients presenting with suspected renal colic is important not only to make the diagnosis but also to assess the size and location of the stone as

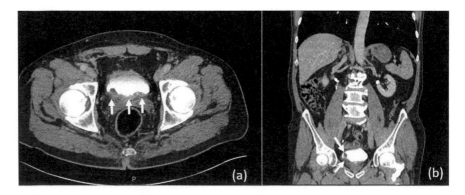

Figure 8.2 (a) Arrows highlight an irregular lesion at the posterior wall of the urinary bladder contrasted against the bladder contrast. (b) The same patient with the lesion marked by arrows in the coronal plane.

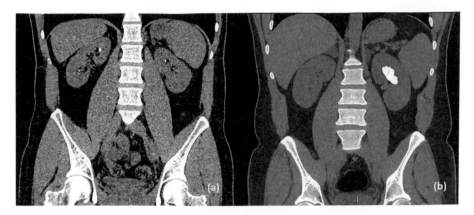

Figure 8.3 (a) Coronal unenhanced CT KUB showing multiple small (<10 mm) renal calculi. These stones do not usually require intervention and are likely to pass spontaneously. (b) Coronal unenhanced CT KUB showing a large (>10 mm) staghorn calculus in the left kidney.

well as to assess the anatomical features of the patient (2,3). Plain X-ray, US, CT and MRI scan are imaging modalities used to investigate patients with suspected renal colic.

Non-contrast CT KUB is the preferred modality with the highest sensitivity (Figure 8.3a). On modern scanners, the radiation dose for these studies is relatively low (comparable to an abdominal radiograph), so in the right clinical context, the study is often justified, even in younger adults.

Accurately describing the calculus size is important as those less than 5 mm in size have a high chance of spontaneous passage, whereas stones greater than 10 mm are unlikely to pass without intervention (Figure 8.3b).

Calcium-based, struvite, uric acid and cystine stones are radio-opaque in the vast majority of cases, although the latter three are usually less dense in terms of the HU than calcium-based calculi. Drug-related stones such as those that arise from administration of indinavir tend to be radiolucent, so care should be taken to look for secondary features of renal colic such as hydroureter and hydronephrosis when assessing the CT KUB of HIV-positive patients taking this medication.

In paediatric or pregnant patients, or those where there is diagnostic uncertainty, ultrasound can be used. Good views of the kidneys and most proximal ureters can be obtained on US, especially in thinner patients. The majority of the ureters, however, are usually obscured, so secondary features of renal colic such as hydronephrosis and absence of ureteric jets (detected using Doppler) in the bladder that suggest an obstructed ureter are relied upon. US can also identify other pathologies that can be differentials of renal colic, such as appendicitis or ovarian cysts.

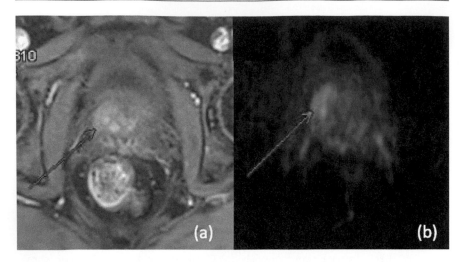

Figure 8.4 Axial MRI images through the prostate. (a) The anatomical information on a contrast-enhanced MRI with fat suppression, the suspected lesion between 9 and 11 o'clock, highlighted by the arrow. (b) Shows the corresponding location on DWI, where the lesion restricts diffusion.

PROSTATIC DISEASE

Plain films have limited use but can detect bone metastases in patients with prostate cancer. CT scan is not used to differentiate diseases of the prostate, but an enlarged prostate may be seen extending above the pubic symphysis on axial imaging, and the volume can be measured above 30 mL on reformatted images (4). Inflammation of the prostate is seen as diffuse hypodensity and enlargement. An abscess may be seen as a well-defined area of hypoenhancement with peripheral enhancement. In malignancy, typically diffuse or focal areas in the peripheral zone where 70% of adenocarcinomas arise, exhibit increased enhancement, particularly in the venous phase. CT scan is also used to assess local and distant spread. MRI is an excellent modality for assessing prostate abnormalities, and suspected lesions are given a score out of 5 according to the PI-RADS criteria; generally speaking, lesions graded 4 or 5 proceed to biopsy. Malignant lesions are typically in the peripheral zone with T2WI hypointensity, focal enhancement and low diffusivity (Figure 8.4a,b).

Both transabdominal and transrectal ultrasound (TRUS) are used to assess the prostate. TRUS is preferred for a more detailed assessment and for guiding prostatic biopsy.

TESTICULAR TUMOURS AND BENIGN SCROTAL SWELLINGS

Ultrasound is the first-line investigation when it comes to imaging the scrotal contents. MRI is considered second line in cases where US is

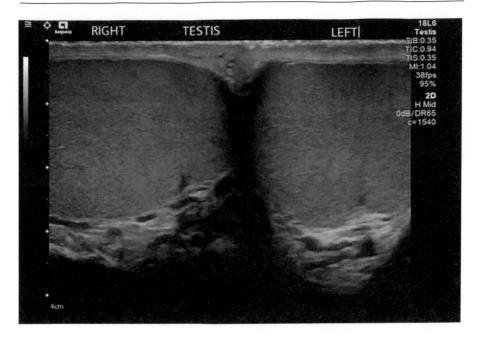

Figure 8.5 Direct transverse US scanning of the scrotum showing the right and the left testes. The testes appear homogeneous and slightly granular. There is no fluid surrounding the testes to suggest that a hydrocele is present.

inconclusive (5). B-mode ultrasound is used along with colour Doppler assessment. CT is used when ultrasound and MRI are not available but is less useful; however, CT is crucial for staging if a malignant tumour is detected. On US, a normal testicle appears homogeneous with granular echotexture (Figure 8.5). The epididymis is isoechoic or hyperechoic compared to the testicle.

Varioceles

Varicoceles are common swellings of the scrotum. The diagnostic criterion of a varicocele on assessment of the scrotum is that the venous diameter is above 2 mm and that there is an increase in the venous diameter in the patient's upright position or during the Valsalva manoeuvre, as well as the presence of reflux in the pampiniform venous plexus. Doppler ultrasound can distinguish among five grades of severity, depending on the level of reflux from the groin down to the inferior pole of the testicle and also the presence of deformity of the scrotum. Idiopathic varicoceles are almost invariably left-sided. The US diagnosis involves the presence of multiple dilated serpiginous tubules posterior to the testis, which may extend to the inferior testicular pole (Figure 8.6a).

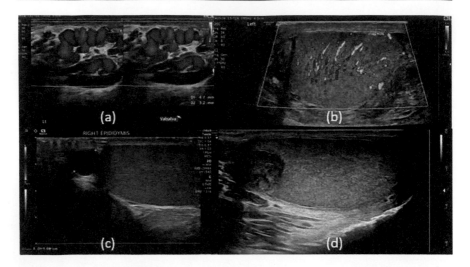

Figure 8.6 US images showing varied pathology of the testes. (a) Dilated vessels in the
pampiniform plexus are in keeping with a varicocele. (b) Granular testis that
contains increased blood flow is indicated by avid colour Doppler signal; these
appearances are typical of orchitis. (c) Benign lesion (cyst) of the epididymis.
(d) Malignant-appearing tumour at the upper pole of the testis.

Orchitis and Epididymo-orchitis

Acute or chronic epididymitis usually causes the epididymis to enlarge and
become hypervascular. In cases of epididymo-orchitis, the testis also tends
to be hypervascular and can be oedematous (Figure 8.6b). The patient commonly also has a hydrocele, which is well seen on US.

Trauma

Ultrasound is used to assess complications of traumatic injuries such as
haematoma, hydrocele and rupture of the tunica albuginea and is highly
sensitive.

Testicular Torsion

For suspected testicular torsion, US can delay surgical exploration and can
yield false negatives as it is possible to detect testicular blood flow in cases of
torsion, which may be an artefact. US appearances are non-specific and can
include a heterogeneous testis and epididymis as well as scrotal oedema and
the presence of a hydrocele. Colour Doppler can demonstrate the 'whirlpool
sign' within the spermatic cord, which has a high sensitivity and specificity
of greater than 90%.

Testicular Tumours

Most extra-testicular lesions are benign (Figure 8.6c) and intra-testicular lesions tend to be malignant (Figure 8.6d). Most tumours are hypoechoic but may be heterogeneous with hyperechoic areas and may contain calcifications or appear mixed solid and cystic. On MRI testicular tumours tend to be low signal on T2-weighted images. CT is used for tumour staging and is not useful for tumour characterisation.

REFERENCES

1. Israel GM et al. Urology. (2005). PMID: 16140062.
2. Renal and ureteric stones: assessment and management. Diagnostic Evidence Review (B) NICE Guideline, No. 118 National Guideline Centre (UK). London: National Institute for Health and Care Excellence (NICE); 2019 Jan.
3. Brisbane W et al. Nat Rev Urol. (2016). PMCID: PMC5443345.
4. Banker H et al. Prostate Imaging. Treasure Island (FL): StatPearls Publishing; 2022. www.ncbi.nlm.nih.gov/books/NBK567721/.
5. Studniarek M et al. J Ultrason. (2015). PMCID: PMC4657400.

Chapter 9

Trauma and Orthopaedics

X-rays continue to be widely used in trauma and orthopaedics as they provide a great deal of bony detail, are easily accessible and can be portable. They are used to assess fractures and dislocations in the trauma setting and also provide diagnostic information when it comes to non-acute presentations such as osteoarthritis and bony lesions. In the trauma setting, it is important to review orthogonal views, which are two views usually but not always taken 90 degrees to one another, as fractures and dislocations can easily be missed if looking at only one view. Certain anatomical locations require special views to allow proper assessment of those particular injuries, for example, the Judet view of the acetabulum of the hip and skyline view of knee to assess the patella. In the context of trauma, it is also important to assess the joint above and below an injury to assess its full extent and avoid missing any injuries. When describing whether a fracture is displaced, the angulation of the distal fragment of the bone with respect to the proximal fragment is considered (see Figures 9.1 and 9.2 for illustration).

Some plain films are labelled by the radiographer with the term 'red dot'. This labelling system was devised in Ealing and Northwick Park Hospitals in London in the 1980s, whereby the radiographer taking the image can highlight any suspected bony injury, especially useful when interpreting the plain film as it increases attention when reviewing the film and reduces the chance of missed injuries in the emergency department.

Depending on the mechanism of injury and with the advent of dedicated trauma centres with CT scanners often located in the emergency department, patients who experience major trauma will often have trauma protocol CT, which will cover the axial skeleton, so injuries such as traumatic spine fractures can be detected with a high degree of accuracy. There is variable coverage of the appendicular skeleton in trauma CT, and limbs may be imaged separately with plain film in the first instance if there is concern regarding fracture, with dedicated cross-sectional imaging performed if a bony injury is detected on plain film. CT is useful as it is more sensitive at detecting small fractures that may not be seen on plain film. CT also enables 3D constructions of any fractures to be carried out, which though not very

 DOI: 10.1201/9781003324362-9

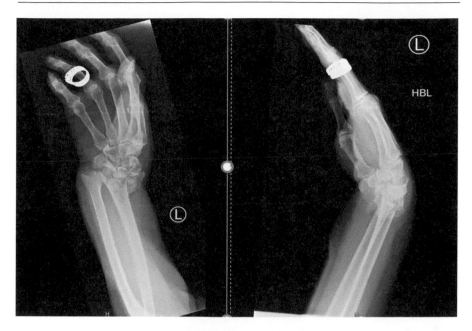

Figure 9.1 Frontal and lateral radiographs showing an impacted comminuted fracture of the distal radius. The distal fracture fragments are dorsally angulated, qualifying this as a Colles' fracture.

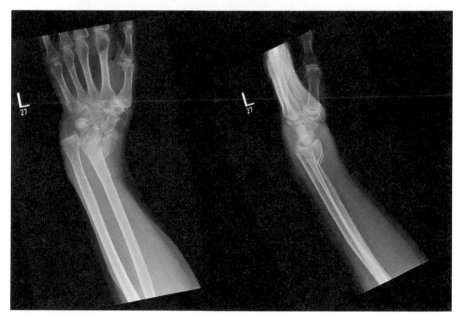

Figure 9.2 Frontal and lateral radiographs showing an extra-articular fracture of the distal radius with volar angulation, known eponymously as a Smith's fracture.

helpful in the majority of radiological interpretations, these can be helpful for orthopaedic surgical planning by the clinicians. Post-operatively, CT is also useful to assess for non-union, which may not be seen on plain film, as well as assessing rotational alignment.

MRI is the best modality to look at the soft tissues, for example, anterior cruciate ligament injury in the knee. It is extremely sensitive at depicting bone oedema, which can be suggestive of fracture in the correct clinical context, as oedema may also be a feature of osteomyelitis or an occult or stress fracture.

Bone scans may be used in certain situations. They can be useful for assessing occult fractures and osteomyelitis, although MRI is often the first-line modality for these conditions. Another advantage of bone scans is that they provide imaging of the whole skeleton. The sensitivity of detecting fractures on bone scan is increased to 95%, at 72 hours after the injury.

Fluoroscopy provides real-time imaging at lower radiation dose compared to standard X-rays. It is portable and its use has become invaluable in the operating theatre to evaluate fracture fixation and placement of implants. As it is a real-time image, the surgeon should be able to interpret the images and needs to understand radiation safety. Although not useful as a diagnostic study as it provides inferior resolution than a standard X-ray, fluoroscopy usually provides enough information to assess fracture fixation.

As well as assessment of soft tissue injuries, US can also aid in detecting fractures by observing for discontinuity of bone cortices. The soft tissues such as ligaments and tendons are well seen on US, and many interventions can also be performed under US guidance, for example, injections of joints with steroids.

FRACTURES AND JOINT DISLOCATIONS

The non-specialist surgeon should be aware of several common fracture complexes, and these are usually well depicted on plain film. The three most common fractures are of the distal radius, the proximal femur (the hip) and the ankle. Along with insufficiency fractures of the spine, fractures of the distal radius and hip are commonly seen in cases of trauma in an osteoporotic, therefore already inherently weakened, skeleton. Osteoporosis is more common in females; it therefore follows that these fracture complexes are also more common in females.

Distal Radius Fracture

This is the most common type of fracture complex. Three types of these fractures are described depending on the displacement of the fracture and whether it is intra- or extra-articular; they are allocated eponyms for ease.

Colles' Fracture

This is the most common subtype of distal radius fractures and is characterised with an extra-articular fracture of the distal radius with dorsal (posterior) angulation (Figure 9.1). There may or may not be an associated fracture of the distal ulna (usually of the styloid process).

Smith's Fracture

This is effectively the 'opposite' of a Colles' fracture as it is an extra-articular fracture with ventral angulation (Figure 9.2).

Barton's Fracture

This is a fracture of the distal radius that extends to involve the articular surface, resulting in disruption of the radiocarpal joint.

Fractures of the Hip

Both AP and lateral radiographs are routinely taken in cases of suspected hip fracture. The important distinction to be made on radiographs is whether the fracture is intra- or extracapsular; intracapsular fractures tend to result in disruption of the blood supply to the femoral head from the medial and lateral circumflex arteries; therefore, these fractures are associated with a higher rate of avascular necrosis of the femoral head. Fractures arising at the junction of the femoral head with the femoral neck (subcapital fractures) and fractures through the shaft of the femoral neck (transcervical fractures) are considered be intracapsular. Basicervical fractures occur at the intertrochanteric region, do not usually disrupt the blood supply to the femoral head and are considered to be extracapsular. Figure 9.3 depicts these areas on a normal frontal hip radiograph.

It follows therefore that an intracapsular fracture (Figure 9.4a) is usually managed with a hemiarthroplasty (Figure 9.4b) and an extra-trochanteric fracture (Figure 9.5a,b) is managed with internal fixation using a dynamic hip screw (Figure 9.6).

Fractures of the Ankle

A number of injuries of the ankle joint can be recognised on plain film. Lateral malleolar fractures are one of the most common types of ankle fractures and are classified using the Weber classification, which aids in management. The Weber classification revolves around the location of the fracture in relation to the ankle joint, and more specifically, the tibiofibular syndesmosis. The syndesmosis is not seen as a discrete structure on X-ray, but its location

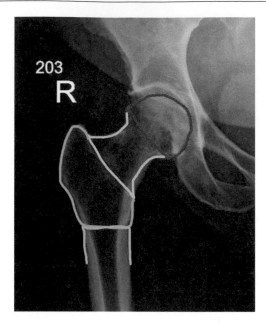

Figure 9.3 Frontal radiograph of the right hip with colour codes indicating the femoral head (red), femoral neck (yellow), intertrochanteric region (green) and subtrochanteric area (blue).

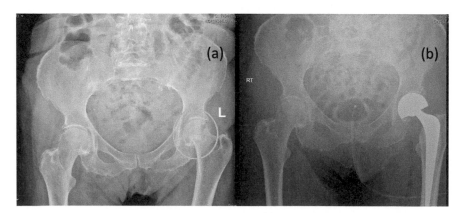

Figure 9.4 (a) A frontal radiograph shows a left-sided neck of a femur fracture (subcapital, caudal to the femoral head at the junction of the femoral head with the proximal femoral neck) highlighted with a circle. Note the foreshortening of the left femoral neck secondary to impaction and disruption of the cortices at the medial and lateral sides of the femoral neck. (b) The post-operative image in the same patient as (a) showing the standardised management of this injury with a hemiarthroplasty.

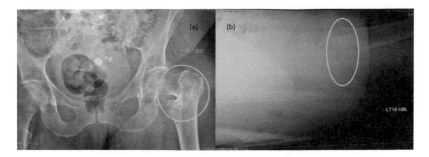

Figure 9.5 (a) Frontal pelvic and (b) left lateral hip radiographs showing a displaced basicervical neck of femur fracture traversing the intertrochanteric region, outlined by the ovals. These fractures are at less risk of avascular necrosis of the femoral head and are therefore managed with internal fixation using a dynamic hip screw (Figure 9.6).

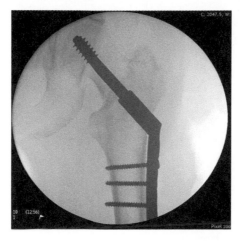

Figure 9.6 Intraoperative fluoroscopic image in the same patient as Figure 9.5 showing reduction and fixation of the basicervical left neck of femur fracture with a dynamic hip screw (DHS).

is effectively at the most distal articulation surfaces of the tibia and fibula. See Figures 9.7 and 9.8.

DEGENERATIVE JOINT DISEASE

Osteoarthritis (OA) is the most common disease of the bony skeleton and is commonly seen in the knees, hips and spine. A number of features of degenerative joint disease can be apparent on plain film (Figure 9.9):

- Loss of joint space, typically because of loss of cartilage
- Subchondral cysts and sclerosis

- Osteophyte formation, typically at joint margins
- Joint deformity, a combination of ligamentous laxity and joint subluxation that happens later in the course of the disease

INFLAMMATORY JOINT DISEASE

Inflammatory joint disease typically affects multiple joints, and the inflammation can occur with the joint, tendons and ligaments and the remainder

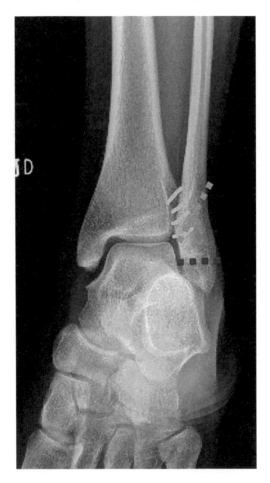

Figure 9.7 Frontal radiograph of a normal ankle. The location of the tibiofibular syndesmosis is highlighted with the yellow lines. Weber A fractures of the ankle occur below the syndesmosis and are often transverse (example of location is shown by red dotted line), and Weber B fractures occur at the level of the syndesmosis and can be associated with fractures of the medial malleolus (blue dotted line). See Figure 9.8 for a description of Weber C fractures.

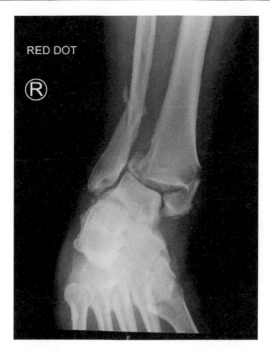

Figure 9.8 Frontal ankle radiograph showing a Weber C fracture. The distal end of the fibular fracture is above the expected position of the syndesmosis and there is widening of the tibiofibular articulation, in keeping with syndesmosis disruption. Note also the fracture of the medial malleolus.

of the periarticular soft tissues. Rheumatoid arthritis and the seronegative arthritides are the most common of the inflammatory arthritides.

Rheumatoid Arthritis

The hands and wrists are the most common joints affected and, in the hands (Figure 9.10), the metacarpophalangeal joints and the interphalangeal joints are the most commonly affected.

On plain film radiography there is soft tissue swelling, joint space loss and eventual erosions.

US and MRI are useful for detecting synovitis and are more sensitive than plain film for detecting erosions.

Seronegative Arthritis

Seronegative arthritis represents a spectrum of diseases comprising ankylosing spondylitis (AS), psoriatic arthritis, reactive arthritis and enteropathy-associated arthritis. These conditions have a commonality of features, most

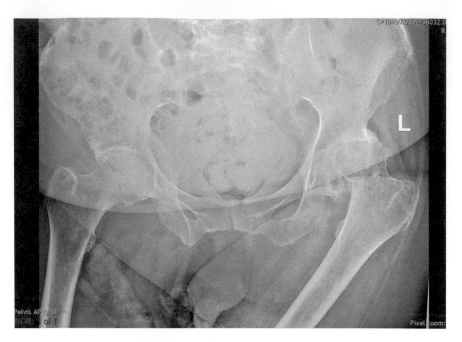

Figure 9.9 Frontal pelvic radiograph showing left-sided hip OA. Note by comparing with the relatively normal right side there is loss of joint space, subchondral sclerosis, marginal osteophytosis and joint deformity.

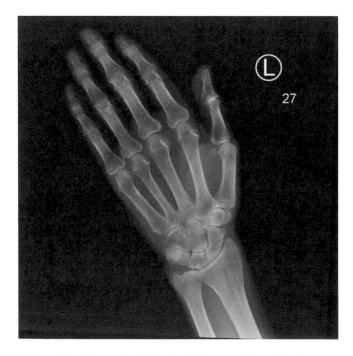

Figure 9.10 Frontal radiograph of the hand showing loss of joint space of multiple interphalangeal joints in a case of rheumatoid arthritis.

usually inflammation at the insertions of the tendons and ligaments. There is also a strong association with the HLA-B27 antigen and a tendency for axial skeleton involvement. MRI is useful earlier in the course of disease where bone oedema synonymous with inflammation can be detected at the insertions of tendons and ligaments. Plain film is useful where bony changes such as sclerosis at the sacroiliac joint in ankylosing spondylitis are established.

BONE AND JOINT INFECTION

Imaging is vital in the investigation of suspected bone and joint infection as early intervention can prevent the long-term devastating effects of chronic osteomyelitis.

Plain films are often performed early in the course of infection, although it can take two weeks for the appearances to change on plain film. Early features of osteomyelitis include soft tissue swelling, periosteal reaction and later bone lysis and fragmentation develop (Figure 9.11).

US is helpful for detecting joint effusions, which can also be aspirated under US guidance for microbiological analysis.

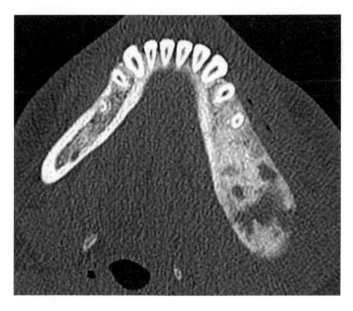

Figure 9.11 Axial CT through the mandible on bony windows showing mixed sclerosis, lysis and fragmentation of the left hemimandible secondary to osteomyelitis.

CT is useful in chronic osteomyelitis to identify lucency, fragmentation (Figure 9.11) and sequestration as well as mapping the extent of disease.

MRI is the most sensitive investigation early in the course of osteomyelitis, with a high negative predictive value to exclude infection.

Osteomyelitis can occur secondary to prosthetic device placement. MRI can be challenging in these cases due to metal artefact from the prosthesis. Serial radiographic interpretation is vital and can show soft tissue swelling and prosthetic loosening. US can be helpful to look for soft tissue swelling or collections around the prosthesis.

Radiology also provides an important role in the management of the diabetic foot. MRI can detect osteomyelitis secondary to diabetic foot earlier than plain film and with greater sensitivity and specificity, but plain film is useful for monitoring and looking for progressive changes. As with other causes of osteomyelitis, the earliest changes are of soft tissue swelling, with development of the triad of osteolysis, periosteal reaction and bone destruction some 10 to 20 days after.

Septic arthritis begins with infection in the synovium that has arisen from haematogenous seeding, with secondary infection of the bone. Joint effusion and synovial thickening inflammation can be detected early with US. MRI is highly sensitive and demonstrates joint effusions, which may or may not be enhancing. In more advanced stages there may be adjacent bone changes, suggestive of associated osteomyelitis. Septic arthritis is confirmed by the presence of positive blood cultures from a joint aspirate that can be obtained under US, CT or fluoroscopic guidance.

SPINAL NERVE ROOT ENTRAPMENT AND SPINAL CORD COMPRESSION

Spinal nerve root entrapment and spinal cord compression are diagnosed on MRI due to the superior soft tissue contrast provided of the spinal cord, cauda equina and exiting nerve roots against the adjacent cerebrospinal fluid (CSF), bone and fat. These conditions can arise from intervertebral disc disease, trauma or lesions such as spinal tumours. Cord or cauda equina compression is a radiological emergency that necessitates urgent scanning.

METASTATIC BONE CANCER

Metastatic bone lesions can be detected on plain film, CT, MRI (Figure 9.12b) and nuclear imaging, for example, on PET scans and bone scans (Figure 9.13).

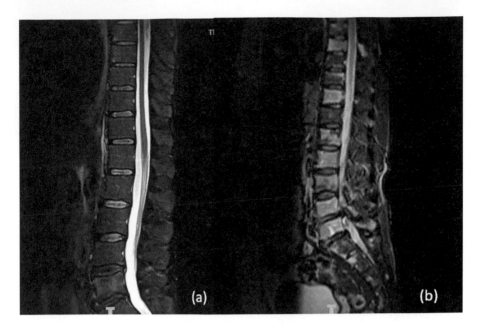

Figure 9.12 (a) Sagittal spine MRI showing no concerning spinal signal. (b) Sagittal spine MRI showing the same sequence as (a) but in a different patient with metastatic disease of the breast. The 'bright' signals in the vertebrae are in keeping with bony metastatic disease.

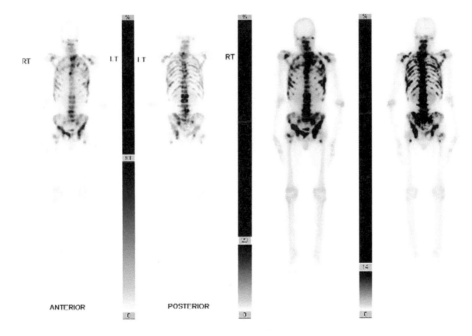

Figure 9.13 Bone scan with diffuse uptake in the axial skeleton in keeping with diffuse bony metastatic disease secondary to lung cancer.

A number of common primary malignancies are recognised to metastasise to bone, including lung (see Figure 9.13), breast (see Figure 9.12b), renal and prostate cancer. Lesions can either be sclerotic or lytic, and they may or may not have a significant soft tissue component. Lesions of the spine can result in cord or cauda equina compression (see above). Metastatic bone lesions cause inherent weakening of the bone and can predispose to pathological fractures.

Chapter 10

Neurosurgery, ENT and Endocrine Surgery

NEUROSURGERY

Intracranial Haemorrhage

Intracranial haemorrhage can either be a result of trauma, hypertension, ruptured aneurysm or secondary to an intracranial lesion. CT remains the first-line imaging modality due to its availability and efficiency, and because acute haemorrhage is inherently of higher density than the brain parenchyma and so can be readily detectable (see Figure 10.1). CT also provides excellent imaging of the skull vault and skull base, enabling any acute skull fractures to be detected in the context of trauma. Haemorrhage can be classified as intra-axial or extra-axial; the former occurs in the brain parenchyma proper and includes brain contusions and hypertension-related haemorrhage. Extra-axial haemorrhage occurs in the subarachnoid, subdural, extradural spaces, or a combination therein. Subarachnoid haemorrhage tends to layer along the sulcal margins (see Figure 10.1) and the lateral ventricles. Subdural and extradural haemorrhage tends to layer along the cerebral convexites, and they can be difficult to distinguish from each other on CT.

The density or the brightness of the haemorrhage alters depending on the age of the haemorrhage (see Figure 10.2). Acute haemorrhage tends to be bright, with loss of brightness with time such that chronic haemorrhages can appear similarly dense to the adjacent CSF. MRI is more sensitive at detecting and characterising the age of intracranial haemorrhage but is not usually performed first line due to the relatively lower efficiency and availability as compared to CT.

Spontaneous intracranial haemorrhage tends to occur in the context of ruptured intracranial aneurysm, hypertension or an undiagnosed underlying brain lesion. It may be appropriate to proceed with MRI to establish if a brain lesion is causing the haemorrhage.

Due to the compartmental nature of the head, when hemorrhage occurs, a mass effect results, which can vary from mild, indicated by effacement of the regional sulci, to gross causing transcompartmental shift such as subfalcine herniation ('midline shift'), well shown in Figure 10.2.

DOI: 10.1201/9781003324362-10

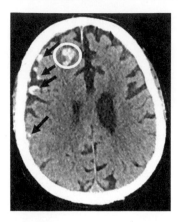

Figure 10.1 Unenhanced axial CT of the head. Bright hyperdense acute haemorrhage layers focally in the right subarachnoid space (arrow). Note
the intra-axial haemorrhage (marked by circle) equating to a contusion in the right frontal lobe.

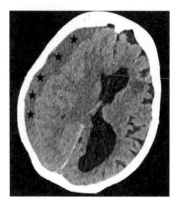

Figure 10.2 Unenhanced axial CT of the head. An extra-axial haemorrhage, highlighted with stars, layers adjacent to the right cerebral convexity.
Unlike the bright intra-axial haemorrhage demonstrated in Figure 10.1,
the relatively low density of the haemorrhage suggests it is not acute.
Note the lack of the normal sulcal definition in the right cerebral
hemisphere. Note also the midline shift is in keeping with subfalcine
herniation.

Space-Occupying Lesions

Due to the closed compartmental nature of the head, intracranial lesions are
also known as space-occupying lesions. Whether they are benign or malignant, space-occupying lesions can result in mass effect, causing detrimental
effects on the patient to ensue. Cross-sectional imaging is crucial as a baseline and for follow-up of any intracranial lesions. CT head is commonly

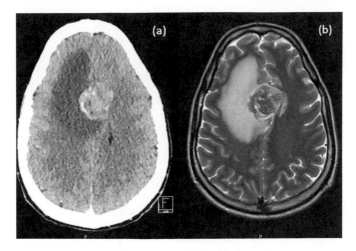

Figure 10.3 (a) Axial contrast-enhanced CT. A large enhancing lesion is present at the midline and is partly surrounded by a crescent of grey tissue in the right cerebral hemisphere, in keeping with the surrounding oedema. (b) Axial T2-weighted MRI in the same patient as (a). The central lesion is largely solid and the crescent of T2 bright oedema shows well on this sequence.

performed as a first-line modality if an intracranial lesion is suspected based on the clinical history and examination because it is readily available and quick to perform (Figure 10.3a). Contrast should ideally be administered in these cases, as this can highlight benign lesions such as meningiomas and malignant lesions such as metastases. Occasionally, malignant intracranial lesions do not enhance because the blood-brain barrier is yet to be disrupted in the course of the disease. In these cases, looking for secondary features on CT such as regional oedema, sulcal effacement and transcompartmental herniation is important.

MRI is more sensitive than CT for the detection and characterisation of intracranial lesions, as various useful sequences can be performed to help establish the nature of lesions (Figure 10.3b). As with CT, administering intravenous contrast can further help characterise the lesion.

Cerebral Abscess and Meningitis

Intracranial infection is usually clinically apparent before imaging is performed, and imaging is usually done to confirm the diagnosis and look for the extent of disease. CT can be helpful in cases of intracranial abscess (Figure 10.4); however, MRI is the preferred modality for this and for meningitis. The latter often yields a normal CT, but the thickened and inflamed meninges are often well seen on MRI.

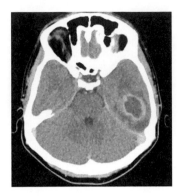

Figure 10.4 Axial contrast-enhanced CT of the brain. A ring-enhancing lesion representative of a brain abscess is surrounded by lower density tissue as compared with the rest of the brain, which is in keeping with oedema. Malignant brain tumours can look similar, hence the need to compare with the clinical history, as patients with neuro-infection are usually very unwell and display infective symptoms and signs.

DISEASES OF THE SKIN, EARS, NOSE AND THROAT

All of the imaging modalities of plain film, US, fluoroscopy, CT, MRI and nuclear medicine have an important role in the characterisation of benign and malignant head and neck disease. The anatomy and pathology of this region is complex but both are very important to understand when interpreting the imaging, as this understanding can prove critical for characterising subtle abnormalities that may have a profound impact on the management of the patient, for example, whether there is extra-laryngeal involvement in the case of laryngeal squamous cell carcinoma (SCC), which would necessitate a laryngectomy rather than medical management.

Diseases of the Skin

The majority of cutaneous lesions are characterised by physicians or surgeons clinically, with or without biopsy. Imaging has a role in the characterisation of cutaneous lesions to determine their extent, particularly in the case of basal cell carcinomas (BCCs) where regional structures such as the underlying bone could be involved. Imaging is also useful in the context of metastatic SCC of the skin of the face or scalp, to determine if there is regional spread to the lymph nodes of the parotid, face or cervical chains. Patients who present with neck lumps could actually have a skin lesion such as a sebaceous cyst, which imaging, namely US, can be used to characterise.

Diseases of the Ears, Nose and Throat

Benign Conditions and Lesions

EXOSTOSES AND OSTEOMAS OF THE EXTERNAL AUDITORY CANALS (EACs)

Both conditions are well characterised on unenhanced CT of the temporal bones. Exostoses are commonly bilateral and caused by repeated exposure to cold water, hence the phrase 'surfer's ear'. Osteomas tend to occur spontaneously and are unusually unilateral. Both conditions may cause narrowing of the EACs that may necessitate surgery; hence, imaging is important to give an overview of the extent of EAC narrowing.

OTITIS EXTERNA (OE) AND NECROTISING OTITIS EXTERNA (NOE)

OE is very common and is usually diagnosed clinically without the need for imaging. If imaging is performed, the lining of the EAC is usually thickened, causing some canalicular narrowing. NOE is a necrotising process of the EAC walls secondary to opportunistic infection, commonly by *Pseudomonas aeruginosa*, that arises in immunocompromised patients. The bony walls of the canal are often eroded, and there can be spread into the central skull base and involvement of cranial nerves, particularly VII, IX, X, XI and XII. Imaging is crucial to make or confirm this diagnosis and for surveillance during and after treatment with long courses of intravenous antibiotics, usually by CT or contrast-enhanced MRI.

OTITIS MEDIA (OM)

This clinical diagnosis is depicted on cross-sectional imaging (CT/MRI) by thickening and retraction of the tympanic membrane (TM), usually with opacification of the middle ear cleft, suggestive of an effusion, often in conjunction with partial or complete opacification of the mastoid air cells.

CHOLESTEATOMA

A differential for OM on imaging, this condition is commonly acquired and causes the accumulation of desquamated skin (the cholesteatoma) in a retraction pocket that has developed, usually at the pars flaccida. The cholesteatoma can cause bony erosion, including of the ossicles (resulting in a conductive hearing loss) and at the roof of the middle ear or mastoid (tegmen), resulting in a dehiscence of the skull base. On CT the opacifying tissue of a cholesteatoma can be similar in appearance to OM, the distinguishing feature being the bone erosion in the case of cholesteatoma. The distinction is sometimes difficult, and in these cases MRI using the specific sequence of DWI (Figure 10.5b,c) can be implemented as the cholesteatoma tissue appears very bright on DWI, whereas inflammatory tissue tends to appear less bright.

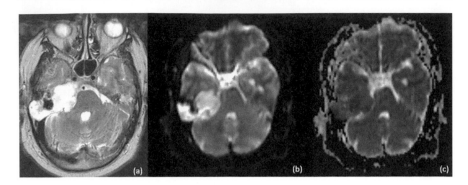

Figure 10.5 Axial MRI images showing a massive lesion of the right temporal bone seen clearly on the anatomical T2-weighted sequence (a). The lesion markedly restricts diffusion as seen by its high signal on the DWI (b) and low signal on the ADC map (c). These appearances are in keeping with a massive cholesteatoma.

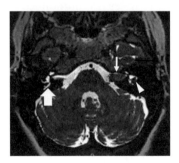

Figure 10.6 Axial heavily weighted T2 image showing obliteration of the CSF signal in the left IAC (narrower arrow), in keeping with an intra-canalicular vestibular schwannoma. Note the block arrow denotes the incidentally dilated right endolymphatic duct (enlarged vestibular aqueduct) and incidental labyrinthitis obliterans in the left semicircular canal (arrowhead).

VESTIBULAR SCHWANNOMA (VS)

The majority of patients presenting with unilateral sensorineural hearing loss (SNHL) will be referred for an MRI of the internal auditory meati (IAMs) to determine if there is an underlying VS causing their symptoms (Figure 10.6). Only approximately 2.5% of the MRI scans are positive for VS, whereas much of the remainder of the patients either have idiopathic or age-related hearing loss (presbycusis). Contrast may be administered when there is diagnostic uncertainty and, in these cases, VSs demonstrate enhancement, distinguishing them from other pathologies such as lipomas.

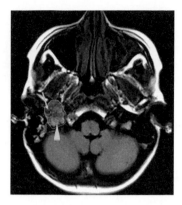

Figure 10.7 Axial T1-weighted MRI showing a large glomus jugulotympanicum out-lined in the right temporal bone. Note the arrow shows a black signal in keeping with intralesional vessels ('pepper'), and the arrowhead shows a bright signal in keeping with an intralesional haemorrhage.

GLOMUS TUMOURS (PARAGANGLIONOMAS)

These neuroendocrine tumours can arise in the middle ear cleft (glomus tympanicum) or at the jugular foramen and secondarily extend into the middle ear cleft (glomus jugulotympanicum). The distinction is important as it helps determine the surgical approach of transmastoid versus the skull base, respectively, and this distinction can usually be made on high-resolution CT or MRI. On CT, these lesions are hypervascular and cause bony erosion, particularly around the jugular foramen in the case of a glomus jugulotympanicum. On MRI, the lesions have a characteristic 'salt-and-pepper' appearance on the T1-weighted sequence, the 'salt' representing intralesional haemorrhage and the 'pepper' representing the filling defects of the intralesional vessels (Figure 10.7).

NASAL AND PARANASAL SINUS BENIGN DISEASE

Most of the pathology detected in the sinonasal system is inflammatory in nature, namely rhinosinusitis and nasal polyposis. Unenhanced CT is the main modality implemented to characterise benign sinus disease as it well-depicts the filling defects caused by nasal polyps and the associated nasal mucosal thickening due to the high contrast provided by the sinonasal air. CT is also indicated to inform the surgeon of any surgical hazards that may be present, including aberrant courses of the anterior ethmoidal arteries and accessory air cells that form borders with the optic canals and the orbits, to aid awareness and surgical planning by the rhinologist.

Benign tumours of the sinonasal system can also be detected on unenhanced CT. These include osteomas, inverted papillomas (IPs) and juvenile angiofibromas (JAs). It is useful to help characterise the lesion and inspect for any specific features of a particular tumour, such as intralesional calcification in IPs and the location at the sphenopalatine foramen in the case of JAs. It is also important to inspect for bone erosion, which may indicate the presence of a more aggressive rather than benign process.

BENIGN SALIVARY DISEASE

Salivary disease is well characterised on US. The majority of benign disease of the salivary gland is inflammatory in the form of sialadenitis, which manifests as heterogeneity in the substance of the gland, which can be due to viral or bacterial infection or due to obstruction of the duct from a calculus or stricture, which are also usually well seen on US. Benign salivary tumours can be diagnosed clinically and confirmed with US, whereby a fine needle aspiration (FNA) can also be performed to cytologically confirm its nature.

Malignant Lesions

The most common primary malignant pathology of the oral cavity and pharynx seen on imaging is squamous cell carcinoma (SCC), with lymphoma coming second in the neck. All three modalities of US, CT and MRI have a place in assessing the primary site and offering staging information about loco-regional and distant spread.

In all cases of upper aerodigestive tract cancer, it is crucial to observe whether the lymph nodes are pathological on the CT/MRI, which is indicated by increased size, necrosis and extracapsular spread (ECS). US is also implemented to assess the nodes, as subtle ECS may be more pronounced on US. US is also useful as the pathological nodes can be targeted for FNA or core biopsy by the radiologist once the diagnostic scan has been performed.

Distant spread is either assessed by CT chest or PET-CT or PET-MRI.

PHARYNX

Nasopharyngeal carcinoma is a virally mediated condition, driven by the Epstein-Barr virus (EBV), hence patients can present at all ages. This tumour can be locally quite aggressive at presentation, whereby the disease can infiltrate the skull base and intracranial compartment; nodal metastases commonly to the retropharyngeal spaces and the posterior triangles (level 5) can also be found at presentation. MRI is the imaging modality of choice as the superior soft tissue detail enables more accurate assessment of the skull base and brain, particularly in cases of perineural spread (Figure 10.8a).

Oropharyngeal cancer is either virally mediated by the human papilloma virus (HPV), typically affecting the younger cohort of patients, or in older patients, it is due to smoking. MRI is the imaging modality of choice to assess for loco-regional disease (Figure 10.8b), as MRI can provide detail of

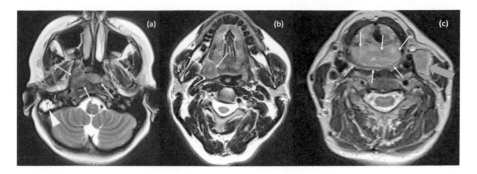

Figure 10.8 Axial MRI images in different patients showing (a) cancer of the hypopharynx, (b) cancer of the right glossotonsillar sulcus (oropharynx) and (c) cancer of the hypopharynx. All the tumours have been labelled with arrows. Note the right mastoid process effusion due to the right eustachian tube being blocked by the tumour in (a) (arrowhead) and the metastatic lymph nodes in the left neck in (c) labelled with a grey block arrow.

small tumours embedded in the tonsillar fossa that display features such as restricted diffusion on DWI. MRI is also helpful to establish if the intrinsic muscles of the tongue are involved when there is disease at the tongue base (important for staging purposes), or if there is involvement of the superior constrictor in cases that will be managed with robotic surgery.

Like the other two subsets of the pharynx, hypopharyngeal cancer is best characterised on MRI (Figure 10.8c), due to the superior soft tissue resolution that is better at characterising if there is involvement of and spread beyond the inferior constrictor, which may require surgical rather than purely oncological management.

ORAL CAVITY

Imaging tumours of the oral cavity are often complicated by the presence of dental metal artefacts, which can interfere with the signal on MRI, causing a blooming artefact that can obscure the region of interest in the oral cavity. As these tumours are often small, direct intraoral US has been used more in recent years to assess the oral cavity, which can give an excellent impression of the dimensions of disease, including the depth/thickness of tumours of the oral tongue, which has an impact on the staging and surgical management.

LARYNX

Small tumours of the vocal cords may be difficult to observe on imaging on account of their size. Larger tumours of the supraglottis or transglottic tumours are often well seen on both CT and on high-resolution MRI, as is a fixed vocal cord. US is also very useful for assessing the larynx, especially when there is a question of whether there is laryngeal cartilage involvement or extra-laryngeal spread through the cartilages or cricothyroid or thyrohyoid membranes, crucial for determining whether the patient may require a laryngectomy for management.

SALIVARY GLANDS

US is often the first-line modality used to assess for suspected lesions of the salivary glands. Malignant tumours of the salivary glands can be very well defined on US, hence why almost all lesions of the salivary glands (except benign lymph nodes in the parotid) should be targeted for FNA. If found to be malignant, MRI is the preferable modality to assess for the location of the tumour and, in the case of parotid lesions, its relationship to the facial nerve.

LYMPH NODES

Patients presenting with enlarged cervical lymph nodes, where there is no primary mucosal lesion, should be referred by the surgeon to the radiologist for a US to assess whether the nodes appear pathological, and if they do, a core biopsy should be performed by the radiologist to establish if the nodes are lymphomatous. In lymphoma, the abnormal cervical nodes tend to be multiple and appear enlarged, solid and often hypervascular. Necrosis and ECS is rare in lymphoma and is more suggestive of SCC metastases.

ENDOCRINE SURGERY

Thyroid Disease

Given the superficial location of the thyroid gland in the lower neck, primary radiological assessment of the thyroid gland is done with US, which provides high-resolution imaging. The most common condition that is identified in the thyroid on US is nodular disease.

Benign Thyroid Nodules

Thyroid nodules are palpable in 3–7% of the population, and nodules can be seen on US in 30–70% of the population. Thyroid nodules can also be found incidentally on CT and MRI performed for another reason. Another advantage of using US to assess the thyroid is the ability to perform a US-guided FNA if cytological assessment is required.

Radiologists use several classification systems to stratify the radiological appearance of thyroid nodules on US, which determines whether the nodules can be dismissed clinically or whether further investigation, in the form

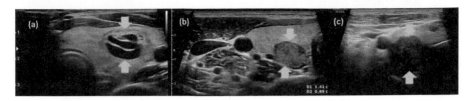

Figure 10.9 Spectrum of appearances of nodularity in the thyroid. The thyroid nodules are highlighted by block arrows. (a) A typically benign-appearing predominantly cystic nodule. (b) A solid nodule which has more indeterminate features. (c) A malignant-appearing nodule, in that the lesion is hypoechoic (dark) with a 'taller-than-wide' appearance.

of cytological assessment with FNA, is required. In the UK, the most common classification system that is utilised is the British Thyroid Association (BTA) guidelines, 2014. These stratify thyroid nodules into five categories, U2–U5 (U1 is no nodular disease), based on their sonographic appearances. The BTA guidelines do not consider the size of nodules in any of their criteria. Any nodules classified as U3 (Figure 10.9b,c) and above should be characterised further with FNA and discussed in the multidisciplinary team meeting.

Benign appearing nodules classified as U2 nodules do not usually require any radiological or clinical follow-up (Figure 10.9a). On US, these appear as well-defined lesions that may be completely or partially cystic. The solid components are often of similar echogenicity to the surrounding thyroid parenchyma and can contain microcysts or colloid, the former appearing spongy/spongiform and the latter appearing as bright comma-shaped foci, also described as a 'comet tail'.

Patients can commonly present with more than one thyroid nodule and each requires sonographic assessment and categorisation. Commonly, the multiple nodules that are present will appear benign and, in some cases, these nodules coalesce to form nodular masses and in severe cases, multinodular goitres. In the case of the latter, it is important to establish if there is any retrosternal component on US, in which case a CT neck and chest may be performed to decipher the extent of the retrosternal component and whether the cardiothoracic service will need to be present at surgical excision to open the chest.

Malignant Thyroid Nodules

Historically, thyroid cancer was thought to be as rare as sarcoma, but with the advent of modern imaging, there has been a dramatic increase in the incidence of papillary thyroid cancer. The overall mortality rate of papillary thyroid cancer has remained relatively static, however, in keeping with papillary thyroid cancer being an indolent condition.

On US, these lesions can appear hypoechoic, with irregular margins, increased vascularity and a 'taller-than-wide' appearance (Figure 10.9c), the latter relating to a larger dimension in the anteroposterior versus the left-right planes. If a malignant nodule is suspected on US, it is important to stage the neck and inform the endocrine surgeon if there are any pathological nodes in the lateral compartment, as this will necessitate an altered surgical approach (neck dissection and thyroidectomy versus thyroidectomy alone if no nodes are pathological).

Thyroiditis

Inflammatory processes of the thyroid are well detected on US. These can be secondary to autoimmune disease or subacute/viral (De Quervain's) thyroiditis. In Hashimoto's thyroiditis, the thyroid appears atrophied and hypoechoic. In Graves' disease, the thyroid is often swollen with a hypervascular 'thyroid inferno' vascular pattern on Doppler. Depending on the phase of subacute thyroiditis, the gland can appear oedematous and hypervascular (acute phase), or contain hypochoic foci (chronic phase), before the inflammatory plaques resolve and the thyroid returns to a normal appearance.

Parathyroid Disease

Sestamibi nuclear medicine scans are an established modality for trying to localise parathyroid adenomas, but the sensitivity of this study is relatively low, especially for smaller lesions. US is a useful modality to search for parathyroid adenomas (Figure 10.10a) but is highly operator dependent in cases

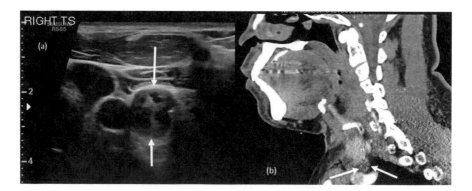

Figure 10.10 (a) A US image of a large right lower position parathyroid adenoma highlighted by arrows. (b) The arterial phase parathyroid CT shows the same lesion in the sagittal section, highlighted by arrows. The thyroid gland lies immediately adjacent to the lesion and is also labelled (THY).

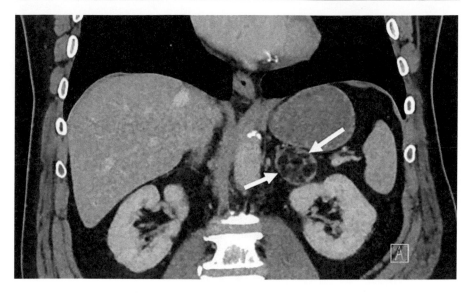

Figure 10.11 Coronal contrast-enhanced CT showing a lesion in the left adrenal gland containing a large volume of macroscopic fat (arrow); these appearances are in keeping with an myelolipoma of the adrenal gland. Adrenal adenomas tend to look more homogeneous.

of hyperparathyroidism. Parathyroid CT has been utilised more recently as an adjunct or substitute for sestamibi scans on account of its increased sensitivity and useful information regarding exact anatomical location, which in conjunction with intraoperative PTH assessment can facilitate a minimally invasive approach to parathyroidectomy, with the associated better outcomes for the patient (Figure 10.10b).

Adrenal Gland Disease

The adrenal glands are well depicted on CT and MRI, and adrenal nodules are commonly seen incidentally on abdominal CT performed for another reason. It is important to use cross-sectional imaging techniques to try and distinguish between benign and malignant conditions. The characteristics such as the definition and the size of the lesions need to be assessed. It is also crucial to measure the density of the lesion, if the density is less than 10 HUs on contrast-enhanced CT, which is compatible with a benign lipid-rich adenoma. If the density is greater than 10 HUs, the lesion should be assessed with dedicated adrenal CT to establish its wash-out characteristics or adrenal MRI to look for the macroscopic fat of an adenoma. Apart from adenomas, other benign lesions that can be characterised on imaging include cysts and myelolipomas (Figure 10.11).

Absence of microscopic fat and or absence of wash-out of contrast is suggestive of a benign functioning lesion (such as a phaeochromocytoma), or of metastasis or primary malignancy. History and biochemical information is vital to aid the interpretation of the cross-sectional imaging in these cases (urine catecholamines test positivity would suggest a phaeochromocytoma, history of malignancy would suggest metastasis).

Index

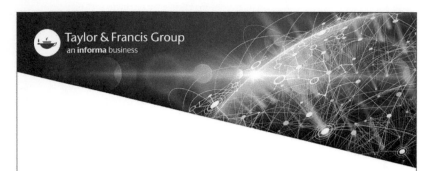